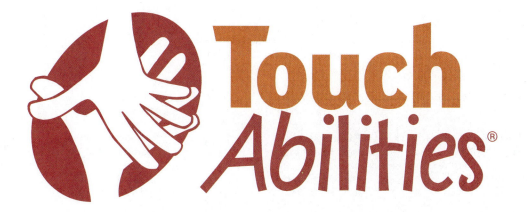

ESSENTIAL CONNECTIONS

Iris Burman, LMT
Sandy Friedland, LMT

Text Design and Composition by Alana Eve Burman
Illustrations by Luc Nisset

THOMSON
★
DELMAR LEARNING

Australia • Canada • Mexico • Singapore • Spain • United Kingdom • United States

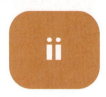

ii

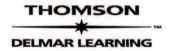

TouchAbilities® Essential Connections
by Iris Burman and Sandy Friedland

Vice President, Health Care Business Unit:
William Brottmiller

Director of Learning Solutions:
Matthew Kane

Acquisitions Editor:
Kalen Conerly

Product Manager:
Natalie Pashoukos

Editorial Assistant:
Molly Belmont

Marketing Director:
Jennifer McAvey

Marketing Coordinator:
Christopher Manion

Production Director:
Carolyn Miller

Production Manager:
Barbara A. Bullock

Production Editor:
John Mickelbank

Library of Congress Cataloging-in-Publication Data

Burman, Iris.
  Touchabilities : essential connections / Iris Burman, Sandy Friedland.
      p. ; cm.
  Includes bibliographical references and index.
  ISBN-13: 978-1-4180-4833-4
  ISBN-10:1-4180-4833-X
  1. Massage.
      [DNLM: 1. Musculoskeletal Manipulations. 2. Therapeutic Touch. WB
535 B962t 2006] I. Friedland, Sandy. II. Title.
  RA780.5.B87 2006
  615.8'22--dc22
                                    2005035325

Notice to the Reader

Publisher does not warrant or guarantee any of the products described herein or perform any independent analysis in connection with any of the product information contained herein. Publisher does not assume, and expressly disclaims, any obligation to obtain and include information other than that provided to it by the manufacturer.

The reader is expressly warned to consider and adopt all safety precautions that might be indicated by the activities described herein and to avoid all potential hazards. By following the instructions contained herein, the reader willingly assumes all risks in connection with such instructions.

The publisher makes no representations or warranties of any kind, including but not limited to, the warranties of fitness for particular purpose or merchantability, nor are any such representations implied with respect to the material set forth herein, and the publisher takes no responsibility with respect to such material. The publisher shall not be liable for any special, consequential, or exemplary damages resulting, in whole or part, from the reader's use of, or reliance upon, this material.

Acknowledgments

We joyfully acknowledge the contributions of our friends and supporters. It is with appreciation and gratitude that we say thanks to Jack Blackburn, Alana Eve Burman, Randy Burman, Kalen Conerly, Sandy Fritz, Ray Infante, Mirka Knaster, Crystal Loiacono, Luc Nisset, Zuriel Nisset, Erica Rand, Linda Riach, Richard Schekter, Ed Wilson, Gina Witt and the staff, faculty and students at Educating Hands School of Massage for their participation in the development, production and organization of this text. We extend a special thanks to the BodyWork practitioners who contributed their expertise in the development of the modalities chapter.

Table of Contents

Linking TouchAbilities® to Modalities Index

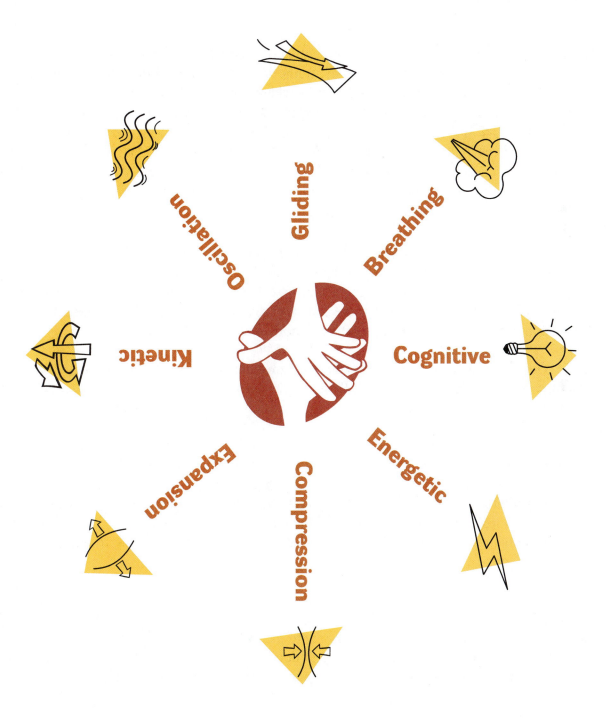

Foreword

As a massage therapy educator who teaches entry level and advanced level students, I have often found myself confused and frustrated when attempting to teach the fundamentals of massage. I personally learned massage in the late 1970s by taking classes in the various modalities popular at the time. There were lots of them, all appearing different on the surface but somehow similar in application. This approach to learning was both valuable and confusing because the language was different for each modality. What I did with my hands and intention were familiar no matter what the course was named or who was teaching it. There reached a point after about 5 years of attending many seminars presented by great educators (and spending lots of money) that I finally realized that there was an underlying theme in BodyWork.

Since those early days the massage profession has evolved, diversified and even become more fragmented. Then, some years ago, something happened. Many "experts in the field of massage" began to identify the more universal and recurring components of massage and BodyWork theory and practice. How exciting it is to be a part of this leap in understanding that, like most things, BodyWork modalities and methods are more alike than different.

In this book, Iris and Sandy have captured the essence of this investigation of thought in an elegant and joyful way. As I read through their simple, yet profound explanation of BodyWork as TouchAbilities®, I am struck by the inspiration, intention and compassion that was put forth to develop it.

I write comprehensive textbooks, so I understand what it takes to concisely explain concepts, theory and skill application. Iris and Sandy accomplish the task. If the main textbooks used in massage education today were compared, there would be and should be a large overlap and agreement about content describing the core and fundamental knowledge base of therapeutic massage. TouchAbilities® captures it all in an experiential manner and taps into intrinsic knowledge of healing touch.

As people begin to learn the theory and practice of therapeutic BodyWork modalities it is important to consider the historical roots of a system to gain a larger understanding of the foundation upon which the system is built. TouchAbilities® does this by tapping into an innate understanding of touch and explaining these concepts in simple generic common language.

This book certainly supports the textbooks I have written and I recommend that TouchAbilities® be used as both an entry point in understanding therapeutic applications of touch as well as an integration text throughout the continuous circle of learning. Learning begins with the simple desire of wanting to know something. As learning progresses, knowledge and practice skills seem to become complex and rightly so. It takes a lot of information, skill and practice to embrace the simplicity of actually understanding what you are doing as opposed to just doing it. During the learning process it seems as if we move though a maze of theory, facts, application, practice and confusion. That's OK—education in general is a bit messy but eventually we come out the other end of the maze owning the simplicity of mastery.

This book describes both a beginning and an end of the learning spiral. Many experts and authors, including myself, contribute to the middle of the learning journey between the beginning and the completion of achieving competency. Each of us contributes an essential aspect of content during the learning journey. Learning never ends and each completed cycle leads to the next entry point for achieving excellence. You can't skip parts—you have to do the beginning, middle and end before moving to the next level. However, the beauty of real understanding is realizing that the entry and exit points of competent professional BodyWork practice are simple, elegant and universal. The strength and contribution of TouchAbilities® to the evolution of BodyWork practices is the joyful and compassionate way it shares these truths.

Sandy Fritz, owner and director
Health Enrichment Center
Lapeer, MI

Preface

Dear reader, if you are like most of us, you know very little about what makes you tick. Scientists explore tangible structure and learn about the chemical, mechanical and other measurable workings of our physicality. However, this is only part of the story. We are much more than this. We are also mind, spirit and energy.

You have a body. But tell us honestly, what do you really know about your body? How do you know what you know about yourself? Did you come with an operator's manual? Did your parents give you a kit with video instructions?

It is our intention that this book take you on an amazing journey of exploration regarding the human body. Buckle up as we move beyond the purely technical and mechanical and take you into the mystery of the body and the magic of touch.

Our Mission

We, Iris Burman and Sandy Friedland, are professional massage therapists. Our mission is to disseminate information and create an environment for others to become aware of the miracle of being in a body. From this perspective, our journey is one of tactile development, structural unfolding and energetic discovery.

We developed the TouchAbilities® curriculum and wrote this book in response to the pervasive categorization and fragmentation occurring in our profession at this time. There are many varied and legitimate schools of thought out there today, but there is no central unifying body of knowledge. We feel that it is important to identify the commonalities and basic guiding principles that are shared by everyone learning *BodyWork* skills, be it students, teachers, practitioners or the lay public.

Our challenge here is to capture in words an experience that is both tangible and intangible. An experience that is multidimensional and complex. It involves subtle and gross sensation, structure, technique, awareness, skills and other elements that exist simultaneously. We have separated the parts in order to teach them. We expect and encourage you, the reader, to integrate and apply them as the unified whole that they actually are.

We have over 35 years combined teaching experience in a massage school, not to mention thousands of hours of individual private practice. We are continually jazzed and stimulated by the opportunity of awakening people to the delight and excitement of conscious touch with caring intent. We train individuals to be present, to touch and interact with others in ways that support balance and maintain optimum health.

This is a learning process of self-discovery that involves consciousness, knowing yourself, understanding your strengths and weaknesses, identifying your likes and dislikes, acknowledging your accomplishments and your ever-evolving phases of physical, emotional, mental and spiritual growth.

What Is TouchAbilities®?

TouchAbilities® is not, in itself, a modality. Rather, it is the basic skillset of touch options— the fundamental ways in which one being can interact with another. These skills can be applied individually but are more usually combined with other skills to create specialized techniques. In our point of view, the skills are the core elements and the techniques are single skills or combinations of skills blended and used simultaneously to support an intended outcome.

A specific collection of techniques, along with a particular philosophical perspective, an identified target population, and/or defined outcome are some of the factors that distinguish a given modality. Each modality is unique, but with close examination it becomes apparent that they are all more alike than different. What's alike is that we're all dipping into the same pool of possibilities. What's different is the individual way in which the skills are expressed.

Understanding BodyWork

Throughout the text we use the term *BodyWork* rather than massage because it is an umbrella term that more aptly represents all aspects of body or somatic therapies: from Acupuncture to Active Isolated Stretching, from Reiki to Rolfing, from Aromatherapy to Zero Balancing, from Eastern to Western, from tangible to intangible. We do use the word *massage* to refer to those therapies that include that term in their own identification, such as Swedish Massage, Sports Massage, Medical Massage, etc.

BodyWork incorporates massage as well as other healing modalities. From the beginning of human history, *BodyWork* as therapy was used for self-care and to assist others. It might have involved rubbing a tired muscle, squeezing a cut, holding an aching belly or nurturing a wounded spirit. This has not changed over time.

Each culture has developed its own particular version of *BodyWork* based on its unique psycho/social/spiritual construct. Touch has been utilized as part of an approach to healing along with diet, nutrition, exercise, meditation, plant medicines and prayer. Historically, techniques evolved that were consistent with the philosophy of a culture. This knowledge was passed down from one generation to the next, first orally and then in written form. Interpretations, translations and further sophistication, influenced by life experiences and society's needs, led to perpetual modification and change.

Intermingling and exchanging ideas between cultures was limited to trade routes and the occasional adventurer. Relative isolation kept the healing practices within a society essentially pure as they were transmitted through the generations. This changed in the 19th and 20th centuries when developments in communication, transportation and other technologies provided instant and distant connection, making the world a much smaller place.

Today, *BodyWork* is an integrated blend of ideas and applications from around the world. It is the sophistication and organization of techniques that reflect humankind's ongoing inquiry and ever-evolving understanding of the body. Specialty approaches are constantly being created as practitioners focus their work on a particular population, situation or condition. Acquiring knowledge through trial and error brings refinement to the vast array of developing systems and approaches.

We define the body as a multidimensional field extending beyond the physical plane. This field incorporates physical, mental, emotional and spiritual essence and integrates anatomy, physiology and energy. This definition lays the groundwork for the term *BodyWork*, which we address from two different perspectives: as an overall profession and as an individual's practice.

BodyWork, as a profession, is comprised of a wide variety of modalities designed to interact with the body in support of balance and good health. As a practice, *BodyWork* is the skillful, intentional application of the techniques of any modality. Both concepts open the mind to a broad picture of what it means to be a *BodyWorker*.

Key Chapters

In the process of writing this book, we sought input from leaders in the field. Their feedback is integrated into the text and featured in chapter 23, called *Linking TouchAbilities® to Modalities*. Here, 32 prominent *BodyWorkers* describe the modality they practice and correlate it to the core elements identified as TouchAbilities® skills. We feel that this chapter powerfully substantiates and exemplifies our position that all modalities emerge from the same primordial soup and graphically illustrates that TouchAbilities® is a unifying model in its representation of universal, common elements.

One of the highlights of our book is SenseAbilities™, an extensive touch vocabulary designed to awaken you to the world of sensation. We've discovered that using a variety of sensorially descriptive words captures experience and gives voice to the felt sense. From depth to density, from color to posture and function...this chapter is absolutely sensational!

How To Use This Book

Because the material is presented in a variety of ways, TouchAbilities® supports a broad range of learning styles. There are symbols, quotes, exercises, and colorful charts and illustrations. The information is delivered in both outline form and narrative description. There are specific definitions supported by synonyms as well as a description of the actions to be taken by the practitioner. To support the integration of skills, each component chapter ends with a list of "experientials," suggested actions designed to guide students to embody the lesson.

This book is richly endowed with engaging visuals that clearly and precisely illustrate the skills presented. In many instances we provide more than one example of how to apply a specific skill. This highlights the nuances inherent in the basic skills and strengthens understanding regarding the flexibility and creativity possible in their delivery. This approach to learning makes it easy for schools to clearly present the basics and then teach students the modalities featured in their curriculum.

Looking Forward

We have come a long way, yet we have barely scratched the surface. Our goal is to revolutionize and integrate the field. We believe that when current practitioners, school administrators and students see the power and simplicity of our book they will use it as a source and reference for change. It is not just words on the printed page; it's about professional transformation. It is a primer, a new alphabet for learning touch. It is a BodyWork education tool designed to develop astute, competent, sensitive, aware and compassionate practitioners.

And this is not the end...it's just the beginning of a movement to globally change the essence and quality of touch education. To create a stronger, healthier, more holistically connected and integrated professional and profession, it is our hope that *BodyWork* schools everywhere will incorporate TouchAbilities® into their curricula as the foundation for skill development. In our experience, students have an easier time learning any modality once they have this initial education and, in the long run, become more proficient, effective, well-rounded therapists.

We are so grateful to the contributors for their interest in, and commitment to, this vision for integration and change. We intend to continue writing and developing this text. It will be an ever-evolving reflection of the processes of the *BodyWork* corpus itself. We invite you to play with us— to contribute, edit, question, etc.

Toward excellence in touch education,

Iris and Sandy

About the Authors

Iris and Sandy have worked together over the last 15 years developing the concepts of TouchAbilities® and the curriculum to support the teaching of it. They have written articles for national and local publications as well as contributed to another textbook on complementary therapies while writing this current text. They teach basic and mastery level courses in both core curriculum and continuing education formats.

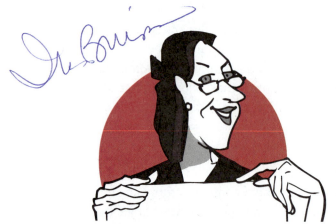

IRIS BURMAN, LMT

Iris Burman is a Licensed Massage Therapist and co-founder and director of Educating Hands School of Massage in Miami, Florida. Her passion in life is to support the personal growth of herself and others. BodyWork has provided a fertile ground in which to do this through her own practice and the sharing of knowledge and skills with her students. She has been a BodyWork practitioner for over 29 years, having specialty certifications in Neuromuscular Therapy, Trager® Psycho-Physical Integration, Sports Massage, and advanced Swedish Techniques. She is most excited about her work in the last 18 years during which she, with the ongoing assistance of her faculty, developed the concepts of TouchAbilities®.

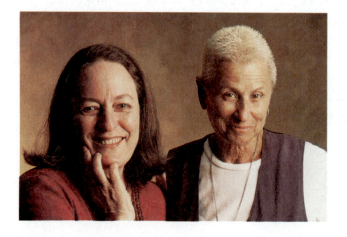

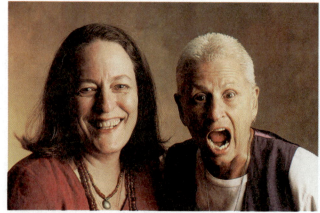

Sandy Friedland

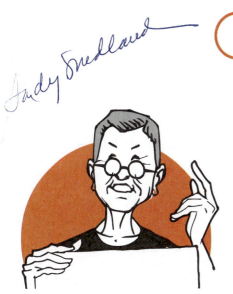

SANDY FRIEDLAND, LMT

Sandy Friedland is a Licensed Massage Therapist in private practice in her hometown, Miami, Florida. She teaches BodyWork at Educating Hands School of Massage and is a creator of the new water _modality_ MDMA, Multi-Dimensional Movement Arts®. She wrote and performed in a Knowledgeware DVD production, "How to Give a Massage." Her approach is spiritual, holistic and eclectic with a specific focus on energetic flow, vibratory frequency and dynamic balancing. She "plays" holographically at a table...on the floor...in the water...using sound, light, oil, color, crystals, essences, balls, magnets, rollers, intention, movement, verbalization and visualization. Her work and teaching explores the mystery of the body and reflects a background in anthropology, philosophy, psychology and the wisdom of Cranial Sacral Therapy, Connective Tissue Unwinding, Polarity, Reflexology, Shiatsu, Trager® and Oriental medicine.

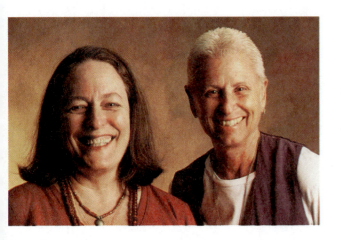
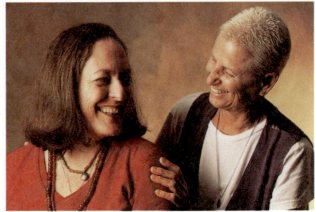

Avi-Khadir Aberman, RPP

SOMA Center
1800 Old Pecos Trail, Suite E
Santa Fe, NM 87505
505-983-2120
avi-khadir@earthlink.net • www.somacenter.org

Avi-Khadir Aberman has more than 25 years of clinical practice and teaching experience in cranial sacral and related therapies. He is founder and director of SOMA, a teaching and treatment center for complementary and alternative medicine located in Santa Fe, New Mexico.

Bruce Baltz, LMT

Deep Tissue Stone Therapy
bruce@dtsm.net
www.dtsm.net

Bruce Baltz is the founder of Spiriphysical, Inc. and developer of Deep Tissue Healing, The Art of Stone Massage. His inspiration has come from working in the fitness and massage therapy industry and experiences as a LaStone® Therapy instructor. His background includes Western anatomical education and Native American healing.

Dale G. Alexander PhD, LMT

2027 Flagler Avenue
Key West, FL 33040
305-393-0929 • 305-296-7339
TROPICAL@aol.com

Dale Alexander has had a clinical Massage Therapy practice in Key West, FL, for 25 years. A teacher and lecturer, he is author of the "Adaptive Mechanisms Concept" and the "Inside-Out Paradigm." These approaches evolved from daily work with clients, personal research, and extensive trainings in Osteopathic Manual Therapy, Soma Bodywork, and Integrated Awareness®.

Mark F. Beck

Cooperative Training Systems
230 North Sunset Street
Fort Collins, CO 80521
970-416-9956 work • 970-493-1427 home
970-472-9522 fax
m_beck@earthlink.net

Mark Beck began his massage career in 1973. He is the author of The Theory and Practice of Therapeutic Massage and Structural Muscular Balancing. He owned the Magic Valley Massotherapy Institute and The Massage Clinic in Twin Falls, ID, from 1980 to 1990 as well as the Cooperative Training Systems from 1995 to the present.

David Allan, DC, CCFC

International School of Integrated Touch
10801 National Boulevard, Suite 607
Los Angeles, CA 90064
310-446-5321
doctorda@gte.net • www.integrated-touch.com

David Allan is the founder and director of the International School of Integrated Touch in Los Angeles, CA. He is a chiropractor and master BodyWorker with years of experience in deep tissue therapy, structural integration, Power Shiatsu, reflexology, trigger point therapy, Reflexatsu, postural education and more.

Ben E. Benjamin, PhD

617-576-0555
Ben@mtti.com

Ben Benjamin is the founder of the Muscular Therapy Institute and a regular contributor to the Massage Therapy Journal, Massage Today, and Massage and Bodywork. He has written several books, including The Ethics of Touch, Are You Tense? and Listen To Your Pain. In private practice for over 40 years, he teaches worldwide.

Jack Blackburn, MTS-SD, LMP, CTP

www.jackblackburn.homestead.com
jackblac@oz.net

Jack Blackburn specializes in body centered spiritual growth and healing. He is a Trager® practitioner, teacher and tutor, a NCBTMB "Class A" instructor and an AMTA national presenter. A Reiki Master, he teaches levels I, II, III and Advanced Reiki for BodyWorkers, and a variety of other classes for care giving professionals.

Patrick Fay, DC

927 4th Street
Miami Beach, FL 33139
305-532-5880
docpfay@cs.com

Patrick Fay practices low force chiropractic, BodyWork, and acupuncture. He has offices in Miami Beach, Key Largo and Big Pine Key. A graduate of Indiana University, Palmer College of Chiropractic, the Oregon School of Massage, and the International Academy of Medical Acupuncture, he studied Positional Release with Leon Chaitow, DO.

Steve Capellini, LMT

www.royaltreatment.com

Steve Capellini has been a massage therapist since 1984. He teaches workshops for therapists interested in adding spa services to their treatment menus, and he consults and trains at spas in the U.S. and Canada. A published author, he is currently writing The Spa Guidebook, a text for use in massage schools.

Sandy Fritz, MS, NCTMB

Founder, Owner, Director and Head Instructor
Health Enrichment Center
204 E. Nepessing Street
Lapeer, MI 48446
810-667-9453 ● 810-667-4095 Fax
healthenrichment@sbcglobal.net

Sandy Fritz has been a massage therapist for nearly 30 years and a massage school owner and educator for 20 years. She is the author of Mosby's Fundamentals of Therapeutic Massage and other texts. Sandy presents continuing education seminars and consults for massage therapy schools on curriculum development and instructional strategies.

Judith DeLany, LMT

NMT Center
900 14th Avenue North
St. Petersburg, FL 33705
727-821-7167
nmtcenter@aol.com ● www.nmtcenter.com

Judith DeLany has spent two decades developing neuromuscular therapy techniques and NMT course curriculum. As co-author of three textbooks and associate editor for "Journal of Bodywork and Movement Therapies" (a peer-reviewed Elsevier journal), her professional focus advances education in all health care professions to include myofascial therapies for chronic pain syndromes.

Jill L. Goldman, LMT, NCTMB

1441 Lincoln Road #302
Miami Beach, FL 33139
305-535-6567 ● 305-282-1918 Cell

Jill Goldman has an extensive background in dance and movement therapies including the Feldenkrais Method®, Pilates and yoga. She has a BA in Professional Administration and is a commercial and fine art photographer. Certified in Postural Analysis, Feldenkrais Awareness Through Movement® and Geriatric Massage, she currently teaches at Educating Hands School of Massage.

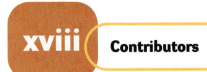

Rose J. Griscom, LMT, Director

Institute of Thai Massage-USA
PO Box 246
Marmora, NJ 08223
609-390-1016
www.thai-massage.org

Rose Griscom is the director and lead instructor of the Institute of Thai Massage-USA, based in New Jersey and Florida. She has been teaching for over 10 years and trains therapists at top spas. Rose leads continuing education workshops approved by Florida state and NCBTMB and maintains a private practice.

Bodhi F. Kocica, LMT

Hoshino Therapy Clinic dba Center for BioTherapeutics
430 South Dixie Highway, Suite 211
Miami, FL 33146
305-666-2243 ● 305-666-9943 Fax
info@hoshinotherapy.org ● www.hoshinotherapy.org

Bodhi Kocica is the director of the Hoshino Therapy Clinic and the Hoshino Apprenticeship Program. Bodhi is the direct disciple of Professor Tomezo Hoshino and brings 28 years of expertise to his work. He is a certified Sports Massage Therapist and AOBTA certified instructor.

Paula Hamelik, LMT

Medicine Cat Enterprises, Inc.
12801 SW 82 Place
Pinecrest, FL 33156
305-238-3646

Paula Hamelik has been a licensed massage therapist since 1992. She was called to study LomiLomi in 1994, and in 2002 was given her teacher's blessing to continue the training lineage, thereby becoming a Kumu LomiLomi herself. Paula currently teaches, and continues to study, the Hawai'ian healing arts.

George Peter Kousaleos, LMT

CORE Institute
223 West Carolina Street
Tallahassee, FL 32301
850-222-8673 ● 850-561-6160 Fax
geo@coreinstitute.com ● www.coreinstitute.com

George Kousaleos has been a practitioner and teacher of structural integration and myofascial therapy since 1979. He contributes to the profession through his active involvement in the development of national certification, massage research, and international sports massage teams for Olympic and Paralympic events. He founded the CORE Institute in 1990.

Kathryn Hansman-Spice, MS, LMT

TRAGER® Southeast Instructor
3580 South Oceanshore Boulevard, Suite 706
Flagler Beach, FL 32136
850-766-0652 ● 386-439-5612 Fax
office@tragersoutheast.org ● www.trager.com
www.tragersoutheast.org ● www.trager-us.org

Kathryn Hansman-Spice is a Certified Practitioner and instructor in the TRAGER® Approach. A Massage Therapist since 1980, Kathryn uses gentle touch and movement to offer new possibilities to the body/mind. She is an experienced educator and school director, specializing in community outreach, bringing touch to special populations from infants to frail elderly.

Bob Lunior, LMT, MSW, LCSW

9180 SW 128 Lane
Miami, FL 33176
boblunior@hotmail.com

Bob Lunior is founder and director of the Shiatsu Institute in Miami, Florida. Bob studied and trained with Wataru Ohashi for six years and was an instructor for Ohashi for four of those years. He also studied Barefoot Massage with Shizuko Yamamoto and incorporates her teachings into his workshops and private practice.

Aaron L. Mattes, LMT, CK

Aaron Mattes Therapy
2932 Lexington Street
Sarasota, FL 34231-6118
941-922-1939 ● 941-927-6121 Fax
www.stretchingusa.com

Aaron Mattes is an international lecturer and a practitioner with over 200,000 hours professional experience. He is a Licensed Massage Therapist and a Certified Kinesiotherapist and has been the clinical director for university sports teams. In private practice for 35 years, Aaron created the system and wrote the book Active Isolated Stretching: The Mattes Method.

Ernesto Ortiz, LMT, CST

Journey to the Heart/Thermo Therapeutics
9199 SW 97th Avenue
Miami, FL 33176
305-632-5603 ● 305-595-1668

Ernesto Ortiz is a facilitator, teacher and therapist who incorporates Bodywork, CranioSacral Therapy, Karmapa Reiki, Integrative Breathwork, Shamanic Healing and the Akashic Records in his work. President of Journey to The Heart, a school with no walls that offers a variety of classes and certification programs, he facilitates numerous seminars and workshops worldwide.

Sheryl McGavin, MBA, OTR/L, CST-D

The Upledger Institute, Inc.
11211 Prosperity Farms Road, D-325
Palm Beach Gardens, FL 33410
1-800-233-5880 ● 561-622-4334
www.upledger.com

Sheryl McGavin is a certified clinician, instructor and international speaker for The Upledger Institute, where she integrates occupational therapy with CranioSacral Therapy. Before that she directed successful private practices in Ohio and Florida, working with pediatrics as well as post-traumatic stress disorder, addictive behaviors and other conditions.

Carole Osborne-Sheets

Body Therapy Associates
11650 Iberia Place, Suite 137
San Diego, CA 92128
858-748-8827 ● 800-586-8322
cos9@aol.com ● www.bodytherapyassociates.com

Carole Osborne-Sheets is an instructor of integrative and maternity somatic therapies throughout North America and the UK. A co-founder of the International Professional School of Bodywork (IPSB), she has been in practice since 1974 and has written two books: Deep Tissue Sculpting and Pre- and Perinatal Massage Therapy.

Julie and Dale McNitt

Bhakti Academe School of Intuitive Massage and Healing
Ophelia's Cottage 146 4th Avenue North
Safety Harbor, FL 34695
727-725-3730
www.bhakti-academe.com

Julie and Dale McNitt developed Bhakti Energy Work™. They have multiple degrees and licenses but their qualifications to do this work could be summed up in one word, *Presence*. They have written the book and produced the DVD called Bhakti Energy Work for Enlightenment.

David Palmer

TouchPro® Institute
584 Castro Street
San Francisco, CA 94114
415-621-6817 ● 800-999-5026

David Palmer began teaching the TouchPro® approach in 1982 and developed the first specialized chair for professional chair massage. He is widely recognized as being the "father" of contemporary chair massage. David studied traditional Japanese table massage with Takashi Nakamura in 1980.

Sharon Puszko, PhD, CMT
DAYBREAK Geriatric Massage Institute
7434 King George Drive, Suite A
Indianapolis, IN 46260
317-722-9896 • 317-722-0511 Fax
spuszko@juno.com • www.daybreak-massage.com

Sharon Puszko, owner and director of DAYBREAK Geriatric Massage Institute, has a private practice, does hospice volunteer work and is an instructor in the Medical Massage Program at the Indiana College of Bodywork Modalities. She travels extensively throughout the U.S. teaching Geriatric Massage Level 1 and Level 2 workshops in massage schools and community colleges.

Richard C. Schekter, MS, LMT, NCTMB
9111 East Bay Harbor Drive, 6D
Bay Harbor Islands, FL 33154
RSneutron@aol.com

Richard has a background in science, as a Marine Biologist and Biological Oceanographer at the University of Miami. Currently a Licensed Massage Therapist and core instructor at Educating Hands School of Massage, he is keenly interested in the effects of massage and is passionate about science and the mystery of transformation in BodyWork.

Linda Riach
Oakworks, Inc.
800-558-8850
lriach@oakworks.com • www.oakworks.com

Linda Riach co-founded Oakworks, Inc. with husband, Jeff, in 1978. The company designs and manufactures products to meet the unique needs of therapists and their clients. As CEO, Ms. Riach has the venue to promote her belief in massage therapy's role in wellness, supporting development and research in the industry.

Fritz Frederick Smith, MD, FCCAc
Zero Balancing Health Association
8640 Guilford Road, Suite 240
Columbia, MD 21046
410-381-9634
zbaoffice@zerobalancing.com
www.zerobalancing.com.

Fritz Smith is the founder of Zero Balancing, a structural acupressure system of healing. Originally a general family physician, he limited his practice for 20 years to Traditional Chinese Acupuncture, Osteopathic Manipulation, and Zero Balancing. He is the author of Inner Bridges, and, soon to be published, Alchemy of Touch.

Jonathan Rudinger, RN, LMT
PetMassage™, Ltd.
3347 McGregor Lane
Toledo, OH 43623
800-779-1001 • 419-475-3539 Fax
Info@PetMassage.com • www.PetMassage.com

Jonathan Rudinger is a Certified Aquatics Leader, and founder of the PetMassage™ Institute in Toledo, OH. He is the president of both the PetMassage™ Research Institute and The International Association of Animal Massage & Bodywork. Author of several books and videos on pet massage, Jonathan presents the PetMassage™ method at dog shows internationally.

Ralph R. Stephens, BS Ed, LMT, NCTMB
Ralph Stephens Seminars, L.L.C.
2287 Holiday Road
Coralville, IA 52241
319-337-6277 • 319-350-1590 Cell • 319-338-6277 Fax
ralph@ralphstephens.com • www.ralphstephens.com

Ralph Stephens is a practicing massage therapist since 1986, author of four textbooks, 14 training videos and regularly contributes to massage publications. He is a continuing education provider specializing in Medical Massage and therapeutic Chair Massage. An internationally recognized seminar presenter, he is regularly featured at state, regional, and national meetings.

Elaine Stillerman, LMT

P.O. Box 150337
Brooklyn, NY 11215
212-533-3188
estillerman@cs.com • www.MotherMassage.Net

Elaine Stillerman has pioneered work with prenatal and post-partum massage for over 25 years. She is the author of MotherMassage, The Encyclopedia of Bodywork and Prenatal Massage: A Textbook of Pregnancy, Labor and Postpartum Bodywork. She developed a professional certification course for pregnancy massage and is a regular contributor to Massage Today.

Pete Whitridge BA, LMT

1232 Bonefish Court
Fort Pierce, FL 34949
772-460-0581 • 772-332-6116 Cell
Pete@floridamassagelaw.com
Pete@floridaschoolofmassage.com
Floridamassagelaw.com
justaskpete@mac.com

Pete Whitridge, in practice since 1989, has served as Chair of the Florida Board of Massage. He teaches "Myofascial Components of Pain" seminars, as well as NMT, Business Building, Florida Law, Prevention of Medical Errors, and Ethics classes throughout the United States.

Lisa VanOstrand

Brennan Healing Science Practitioner
Doctor of Medical Qigong
786-512-7096
lisavano@webspan.net
www.lisavanostrand.com

Lisa VanOstrand, is currently the Dean of Advanced Studies at Barbara Brennan School of Healing where she has taught since 1995. She earned her doctorate in Medical Qigong from China and is a certified Core Energetics Therapist and certified yoga teacher. Lisa's private practice includes long-distance healings.

Ed Wilson, PhD, LMT

Educating Hands School of Massage
120 SW 8th Street
Miami, FL 33130
305-285-6991 extension #303
edreflex@aol.com

Ed Wilson is a Licensed Massage Therapist/Certified Reflexologist active in the Reflexology Association of America and the International Council of Reflexologists. Ed directs a 100-hour certification program in Reflexology, presents Reflexology seminars at various spas in Florida and the Bahamas, and teaches massage classes at Educating Hands.

James Waslaski, LMT

The Center for Pain Management
3107 Riverbend Drive
Hurst, TX 76054
800-643-5543

James Waslaski, author, international lecturer and teacher, has pioneered deep, pain-free orthopedic and medical massage techniques for the treatment of chronic pain and sports injuries. He has over 20 years of experience working with the medical profession as well as professional and Olympic athletes. James has produced a series of video-tapes and published articles in magazines worldwide.

Yamuna Zake

YAMUNA® (studio name)
132 Perry Street
New York, NY 10014
www.yamunabodyrolling.com • www.yamunastudio.com

Yamuna Zake began developing Body Logic in 1980. Based on the principles of Body Logic she created Body Rolling to enable people to take care of their own bodies. The work continues to evolve as she practices and teaches. Today there are over 700 trained Body Rolling practitioners throughout the United States, Canada and abroad.

Navigating Through This Book

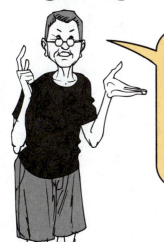

Use this information nonlinearly...

Everything is connected. Everything connects. Be sure to mix and match.

Create, deconstruct and recreate your own relationship to the concepts presented in this book.

The heart of our book is about the *skills* of TouchAbilities®. To promote learning these *skills*, they are organized into groups called *Components*. Each *Component* is featured in its own chapter. There is a basic discussion of each category to present the philosophical basis for our organization.

To support a variety of learning styles, each *skill* within a *Component* includes the following:
1. Definition to clarify use and meaning
2. Synonyms to highlight the nuances of the *skill*
3. Intentions, as application options, listed in outline form for easy reference
4. Practitioner's actions to clarify the physical, mechanical aspects of each *skill*
5. Narrative to expand the definition and discuss the purpose for, and application of, the *skill*
6. Illustrations to demonstrate the application of the *skill*

Each *Component* section concludes with a listing of some of the *modalities* that incorporate the *skills* of that *Component* as an integral part of their system. More detailed information and charts, correlating the *techniques* used by a given *modality* with the TouchAbilities® *skills*, are featured in chapter 23.

The *SenseAbilities*™ chapter introduces a sense vocabulary that is intended to promote sense awareness for both practitioner and client. Each term, word or phrase is meant to conjure up images that become references for communication.

Italicized words that appear throughout the text are defined and listed in the Glossary.

part

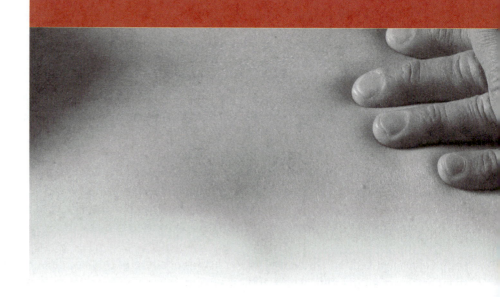

TouchAbilities® Fundamentals

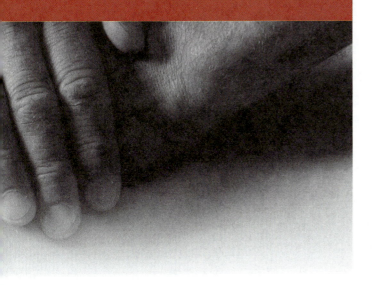

chapter

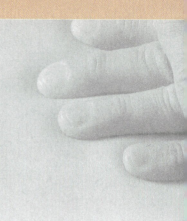

BodyViews

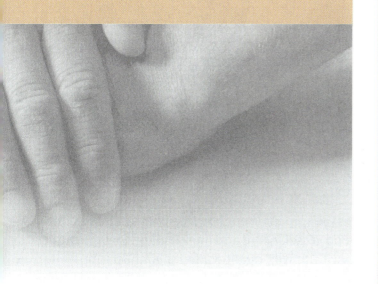

BodyViews

Introduction

There are hundreds of *BodyWork* modalities, most of them are variations on similar themes. Each *modality* is organized around a *general* approach through which to "see" the *body*; in other words, *BodyViews*. *BodyViews* represent a conceptual framework that makes it easier to grasp today's vast variety of *BodyWork* approaches and *techniques*. The categorization of these philosophical and the-oretical "views" is inspired by the ideas presented in Mirka Knaster's book, <u>Discovering the Body's Wisdom</u>. They are: the Structural View, the Functional View, the Movement View, the Energetic View and the Convergent View.

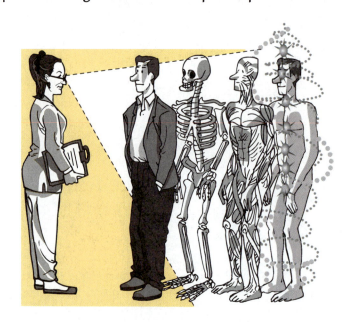

Structural View

The **Structural View** is based on the *paradigm* that the way in which a *body* is held in gravitational space is indicative of its response to physical, mental and emotional stimuli. Structuralists use an "art of seeing" to observe and assess the signs of fascial support inherent in the relationship between flesh, bones and the pull of gravity.

Fascia is a flat membrane of tough connective tissue spread throughout the *body* in a three dimensional web. It surrounds every organ, bone, blood vessel, nerve and muscle right down to the cellular level. A plastic, highly adaptive material with tensile qualities, *fascia* connects, separates, defines and binds everything from head to toe and allows the *body* to retain its shape. Because *fascia* is everywhere and touches everything, whatever happens to any one part of the *body* has an effect on every other part. The goal of a structural *BodyWorker* is to optimize and maintain efficient verticality by freeing restrictive holding patterns within fascial planes. Structure influences form and function.

Functional View

The **Functional View** is based on the *paradigm* that our personal style of movement is learned and that these movement patterns are held within our neuromuscular system. With intention, we can create efficient and economic movement that will more optimally serve us. It is important to become aware of inherent patterns, and select *body* parts and movement strategies that support sensorimotor reeducation. Functionalists look at posture, strength, range and quality of movement, to provide guidance and opportunity for action, using the least amount of effort and energy. Function affects structure.

> **BodyViews- A general approach through which to "see" a *body***
>
> - **Structural View**
> - **Functional View**
> - **Movement View**
> - **Energetic View**
> - **Convergent View**

Movement View

The **Movement View** is based on the same *paradigm* as the **Functional View,** yet takes a different form of expression. It focuses on individual or interactive movement within an organized system such as dance, yoga or martial arts. Used therapeutically, the *modalities* within this view, as in the **Functional View**, take one on a journey of kinesthetic awareness and self-sensing, to discover new possibilities and more effective movement patterns.

Energetic View

The **Energetic View** is based on the *paradigm* that we have a deep and abiding relationship with energetic forces inherent in the universe. In this view the basis of our existence is our connection to, and reflection of, this energy. The therapeutic goal of a *modality* within this view is to establish and maintain an uninterrupted flow of this universal life-force energy to support balance. Each *modality* presents a theory regarding the manner in which energy moves through the *body*. These systems identify energetic pathways, flows, channels, zones, points and pulses, and introduce *techniques* to influence them.

Convergent View

The **Convergent View** is based on the *paradigm* that experiences and emotions are held in the *body* and, over time, the associated energy is expressed in the physical form. In other words, the *body* is shaped by experiences. These are *body*-oriented therapies, not psychotherapies. They emphasize the somatic *component* of posture and movement while addressing the mental and emotional manifestations in living tissue. By bringing awareness to specific areas through dialogue, physical contact and positioning, one can consciously resolve "physical manifestations of emotional issues or emotional expressions of physical issues" (Knaster, 1996). The systems in this view focus on personal revelation and understanding that leads to transformation and new options for expression and behavior.

chapter **2**

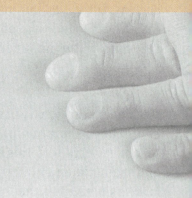

Historical
Development

"No one technique is the sure-fire answer for all people under all conditions. Some people get lasting relief from chiropractic or acupuncture, while others do not. Some people get the results they need from only one body therapy, while others mix several approaches because they build on or complement each other.... There are infinite varieties, and you will work out your own sequence. Success has less to do with what's 'right' and more to do with what's right for you and at what time...."

Mirka Knaster,
Discovering the
Body's Wisdom, 1996

Historical Development

Introduction

Most *modalities* emerged out of an individual quest to solve a personal problem. Challenged to find an answer for an existing situation or issue, people like Per Henrik Ling, Moshe Feldenkrais, Ida Rolf and Milton Trager were compelled to explore options for persistent health concerns. Their search led them to look beyond existing practices that did not offer them solutions. They were asking new questions. By challenging the edges of the known they discovered new ways of "looking" that provided effective intervention *techniques*. Excited by their own discoveries, they started sharing their experiences with others. Their personal stories grew into a context for relating to the *body*. *Modalities* were born. Schools developed to train others in the practice of these touch *skills*.

Swedish Massage

Essentially, modern Western *BodyWork* practices originated in Europe in the 19th century and are based on *skills* developed by Per Henrik Ling, who laid the groundwork for Swedish Massage. Ling's work was popularized by Johan Mezger in the mid-1800s and brought to the U.S. by the brothers Charles F. and George H. Taylor in the mid- to late 1800s. Swedish Massage features the *techniques* of effleurage, petrissage, friction, vibration, tapotement and joint mobilization. Most contemporary schools base their core curriculum in alignment with this Swedish thinking and classification of *techniques*. However, very few limit their training to these six applications. They go beyond them and present *techniques* other than those founded in Ling's work. Blending and cross-fertilizing created derivatives of classic Swedish that are most commonly taught and currently practiced in the United States.

21st Century BodyWork

Twenty-first century *BodyWork* is a compilation of "the best of" whatever happened prior to the year 2000. The evolutionary journey and developmental process of understanding the *body* has moved from the concrete physical to once again include the invisible world of energetic flows and dimensions. Sophisticated technology continually reveals information that expands awareness of what it means to be alive. Practitioners are constantly exploring new realms, learning new ways to improve and maintain *homeostasis*— well-being and good health.

Twenty-first century *BodyWork* is cutting edge. Therapists are pushing the envelope on definitions and traditional notions of touch and concepts of what is being touched. Flesh is more than tissue; anatomy is more than structure; physiology is more than function. Current practice recognizes that the interaction of all the elements is more dynamic and vast than our historical and even our present-day understanding.

Global Fusion

What developed over the last 180 years in private practice, spas, resorts, health clubs and medical centers throughout Europe and the U.S. appears today alongside and integrated with *BodyWork* approaches from the East and healing traditions of indigenous populations from around the world. This global fusion has created the need to identify the broader ground that forms the philosophical and technical basis for the multitude and variety of touch *modalities* available today.

TouchAbilities® provides such a ground.

chapter **3**

TouchAbilities® Essential Connections

TouchAbilities® Essential Connections

Introduction

TouchAbilities® are the fundamental ways of interacting with and/or acting upon and between *bodies*. Developed from years of teaching and professional experience, this foundational approach to *BodyWork* identifies and organizes 26 specific *skills* in eight categories. These *skills* incorporate physical manipulation of soft tissue as well as dynamic interaction with the *body's* mental and energetic *fields*.

The elements of TouchAbilities® are introduced here in a specific order—an intentional progression for learning purposes only. In practice, however, the challenge for the practitioner is to creatively blend the *skills*. TouchAbilities® is nonlinear. It is an ever-changing, ongoing, integration of combinations and recombinations. There is no numeric sequence, no "right" order, no fixed system. TouchAbilities® *skills* are the building blocks of the touch *modalities*.

Each of the eight categories, known as Components, represents a set of skills with common characteristics and shared purpose in relation to the body. The Components are as follows:

Breathing Component
Cognitive Component
Energetic Component
Compression Component
Expansion Component
Kinetic Component
Oscillation Component
Gliding Component

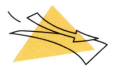

Gliding
sliding/planing
rubbing

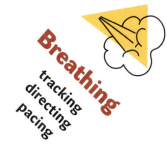

Breathing
tracking
directing
pacing

Oscillation
vibrating
shaking
striking

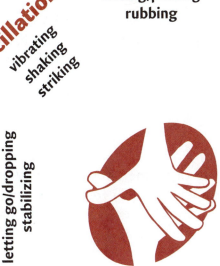

Cognitive
visualizing
inquiring
intending
focusing
transmitting

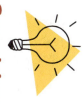

Kinetic
holding/supporting
mobilizing
letting go/dropping
stabilizing

Energetic
sensing
intuiting
balancing

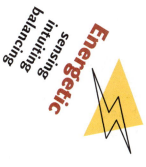

Expansion
pulling
lifting
rolling

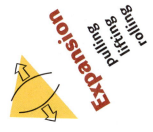

Compression
pressing/pushing
squeezing/pinching
twisting/wringing

"...we are a multi-dimensional creation with coexisting 'bodies'.... Our physical body is composed of matter; our subtle body is energy, thought and emotion; and our causal body is a spiritual source of energy. Health is the integration of all aspects of our being."

Mirka Knaster,
Discovering the Body's
Wisdom, 1996

"How alive we are, how deeply responsive and expressive we are, shows in the graceful shape of our body, which reflects our connectedness of feeling, thought and action.... How we live our bodies is the story of our process."

Stanley Keleman,
Your Body Speaks Its Mind,
1975

Essential Connections

Applying TouchAbilities® is an experiential process, an "in the moment" dialogue between *bodies*. It is a conversation (verbal and nonverbal) used to recognize and connect with the current *state* of an individual. It can be used to identify areas where actions, *waves* and/or flows are obstructed and/or distorted, and to apply *techniques* that re-establish a more functional dynamic.

Dysfunction and pathology, however, are not the sole rationale for *BodyWork*. A person in good health will benefit as well. A therapist might focus anywhere on a healthy *body* with an intention to "push the envelope," polish and further refine an existing *state* of balance. This may support optimal function, improve performance and promote a sense of well-being.

The use of these essential *skills* provides multiple avenues for connection. One can give a treatment to someone, receive a treatment from someone or work on themselves. The relationship between client and therapist, no matter which role you play, is reciprocal. One does not touch without being touched. In the process of learning to assist others through *BodyWork*, TouchAbilities® can serve as a valuable tool for "self" discovery. It is through constant personal exposure to the power and potential of these *skills* that a therapist can most competently and effectively learn to guide others. Receiving a *BodyWork* session is as essential to learning as giving one.

We define the *body* as a *multidimensional field* that extends into the space beyond the physical. It is an organized dynamic of material substance integrating with energy *fields* incorporating physical, emotional, mental and spiritual essence.

TouchAbilities® is also *multidimensional*. What lives through and beyond *technique* is possibility- intention- the experiential value of relationship.

Energy manifests on the physical plane as internal and external *waves*. It includes the inner *waves* of respiration, circulation, digestion, elimination and thought, and the outer *waveform* influences of light, sound, water, weather, earth changes and cosmic shifts.

In *BodyWork*, the *bodies* of the practitioner and client interface in the *field of engagement*. This space of connection offers a window into current internal and external *states*, allowing for intentional therapeutic exchange. Essentially, a therapist uses TouchAbilities® to explore patterns in material and energetic *fields*, interacting with *waves* and reverberations, to establish balance and enhance vitality and wholeness.

"We not only can experience nature in terms of particle (form and structure) and the wave (movement and vibration), but can also experience the interface where they meet- standing in a strong wind, leaning into a tree, or at any interface where movement meets form."

Frederick Smith, M.D.,
Inner Bridges, 1986

"Touch is our first language... Touch is our one reciprocal sense. We cannot touch another without being touched ourselves."

Clyde Ford,
Where Healing
Waters Meet, 1989

chapter **4**

Presence

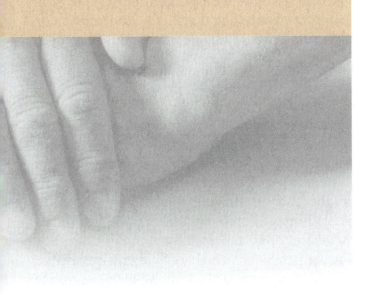

Presence

Jack Blackburn

Introduction

There is a *state* that most of us are trying to create without really knowing it, a *state* that takes us out of tension, confusion, and doubt, a *state* that is so common, that there is no time and no place when it is not available to us. The *state* we're referring to is *presence*. And yet, we spend less time being consciously present than any other activity we perform, mentally or physically.

As *BodyWorkers*, we can choose to become present for longer and longer periods of time. We can teach our clients to be aware of the *state* of *presence*; and together we can, moment by moment, reap the benefits of fully clear conscious awareness.

Body Systems

The *body* is designed with intricate systems and networks that support us for many years. The nervous, digestive, respiratory, immune and other systems operate continuously with or without our conscious involvement. As with any organism, aging causes the system to become less resilient and less responsive to challenge and change. However, *BodyWorkers* know how each system is affected by their own and their client's *state of being*. When we feel open and enthusiastic about our lives, these systems seem to function highly efficiently. Sadness and negative attitudes depress and compromise them; worry and cynicism produce premature aging.

Body Language

BodyWorkers are uniquely positioned to learn the language of the *body* in extraordinary ways. We get to directly monitor it qualitatively and quantitatively by using our hands and minds. We enter a place of continuous awareness of our clients' bodily systems and responses: breath, blood circulation, reflexive reactions, tissue tonus and connectivity, degrees of aliveness

> "Presence is the movement toward stillness in the midst of chaos, the capacity to include conflict in our experience without rejecting it. Presence implies a sophisticated balancing act between extremes of mood, emotion, sensation and thought. This intention involves a quality of mindfulness. Mindfulness simply means that we pay attention, we watch or track our body/mind experience. We attend to the moment-to-moment nature of our ongoing experience."
>
> Michael Shea,
> Somatic Psychology
> For BodyWorkers, 1996

and vitality, peristalsis, *palpation* of deep organs, and relaxation effects. We can feel changes through our hands often before the client becomes aware of them. When we are focused enough in our work, we not only feel the changes that are occurring for our clients, we can also experience changes in our own *body*.

As we become more *skilled*, we are able to work with these responses more consciously to help change the client's *state* of being, no matter what brought them to us in the first place. The way that we most effectively develop this sensitivity is to become fully present to what we are experiencing as we interact with our clients.

Present Moment

Our bodies only exist in the present moment. This existence, on the physical plane, is reliant on healthy function of the body's vital systems. It is also highly influenced by our emotions and thoughts. We pay more attention to the vital systems than to how our *state* of awareness and that of our client, affects those systems and vice versa. When we make a conscious choice to link our knowledge of the *body* with *presence*, we take our work and our profession further than we can imagine.

Systems in the *body* are linked to the present moment; the sensations we feel are also linked to the present moment, meaning that they only occur "now." If we pay attention, we will find that every thought, every emotion, every action, and every *body*-regulated

Axioms that relate to living in the present moment:

- The *body*, although certainly a product of the past, exists only in the present moment

- The *body* is a two-way communication medium between itself and the environment

- The *body* never lies

- The *body* is a living reflection of where our inner and outer lives intersect

- There is a footprint of every step we have ever taken, physically, mentally emotionally and spiritually, recorded in the *body*

- Presence allows us direct access to those footprints

system produces sensations. And, when we consciously choose to monitor these sensations in our clients' bodies, as well as our own, we open incredible new doors of perception and awareness.

Mindfulness

Almost every spiritual tradition teaches some form of *presence* or mindfulness. Every type of *BodyWork*, whether mechanically, somatically or energetically based, gives us conceptual tools for connecting with, and influencing, the various systems of the *body*. When we add the power of *presence* to those concepts and understandings, our work becomes deeper and more meaningful.

There are many ways to achieve *presence* and to bring our clients to the same *state*. For example, when we stay in present time, focusing on the momentary and ongoing sensations in the *body*, we create a place of clarity. Recorded in the *body* is a footprint of every step we have ever taken - physically, emotionally, mentally and spiritually. *Presence* allows us direct access to those footprints.

"Mindfulness means paying attention in a particular way: on purpose, in the present moment, and non-judgmentally. This kind of attention nurtures greater awareness, clarity, and acceptance of present-moment reality. It wakes us up to the fact that our lives unfold only in moments.... To cultivate mindfulness, you may have to remember over and over again to be awake and aware. We do this by reminding ourselves to look, to feel, to be. It's that simple...checking in from moment to moment, sustaining awareness across a stretch of timeless moments, being here, now."

Jon Kabat-Zinn,
Wherever You Go,
There You Are,
1994

Body
Mechanics

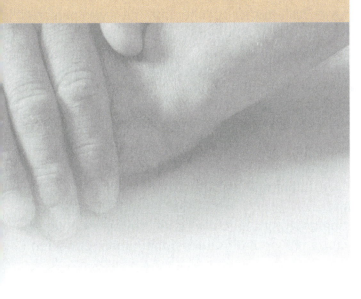

Body Mechanics

Introduction

For our purposes, *body mechanics* is the efficient use of the *body's* energy and physical structure in the performance of a task. "Good" *body mechanics* is an art, a seamless flow of combinations of posture, balance, direction, locomotion, stillness, strength, intention and angle. It is the manifestation of a *body* in motion, poised and powerful in alignment, awareness and actuation. It involves an intricate *feedback loop* of sending and receiving, all the while using the *body* in a way that maximizes the intent/experience for both the therapist and the client. You not only sense response and reaction, you become response and reaction. The *body* is an amazing entity that monitors and modifies whatever it initiates. While you are *in* a process, you *are* that process. Nothing within us changes without our participation. We're already involved so we may as well be conscious about it.

The unique combination of structure, strength, flexibility and energy in each *body* allows for infinite variations in an individual's expression of good *body mechanics*. Inherently it is a very personal matter. Effective *body mechanics* supports the therapist to use less energy, establish clearer lines of nonverbal communication, better respond to client's needs, and experience for themselves the energizing effects of *BodyWork*. Bottom line, it enhances the quality of any *BodyWork* session.

Effective body mechanics supports therapist to:

- **Use less energy**

- **Establish clearer lines of nonverbal communication**

- **Better respond to client's needs**

- **Experience for themselves the energizing effects of BodyWork**

- **Enhance the quality of any *BodyWork* session**

Body mechanics is not just placing the back foot a certain way or relaxing the shoulders or softening the knees. These are important physical behaviors, but thought and intention play a vital role as well. Ultimately, delivering/applying a touch *skill* is an intricate expression of simultaneous multidimensional interconnected processes.

Proprioception is a big factor in efficient, effective, effortless *BodyWork*. It keeps us conscious of where we are in space, how much pressure we can exert and at what speed we can operate without falling over or straining ourselves. *Proprioception* also guides us in determining what angles we can use to come in toward or pull away from the client and consistently stand in our strength.

Developing good *body mechanics* is a very unique and personal process. Here are some concepts and guidelines for practitioners to use in discovering and developing their best form. We encourage therapists to use and modify this list as needed to support specific intentions and situations.

- Center and balance your energies prior to, and throughout, a session
- Be conscious of, and use, your breath to enhance the work
- Adjust table height to accommodate your *body*, the client's *body* and the task at hand
- Face your *body* in the direction you are working or moving toward, i.e., feet and hips and trunk and head
- Stack head and trunk over pelvis for vertical alignment with gravity
- Relax shoulders, arms, hands and knees
- Keep wrists as straight as possible (avoid hyperextending or hyperflexing the wrist or any other joint)
- Position the client's *body* for easy access and to avoid overreaching
- Source power from the *ground points* (e.g., feet) and deliver power through the contact points (e.g., hands)
- Deliver power via the whole *body*
- Pour power from one *ground point* to another when moving through space

If your work requires leverage and subsurface connection, consider these additional strategies:

- Extend arms away from the trunk, maintaining elbows in a soft (slightly bent) position
- Maintain hips under or slightly behind shoulders
- Use *body* weight, rather than muscle strength, to deliver power

Other helpful strategies:

- Train your nondominant side and equalize the use of your *body*
- Exercise and stay fit
- Stay hydrated by drinking adequate quantities of water
- Use a carrying aid (bag or wheels) when transporting your table and other supplies
- Receive good *BodyWork* regularly

Power and Force

In creating graceful, efficient, effective movement it is critical to become aware of the mechanisms for power and force. Power is the potential to exert effort for a purpose; it is the capability of acting or producing an effect. It can be intangible, such as mental or emotional power, or tangible, such as that created by muscular activity. Force, in this context, is the expression of power delivered through the physical *body*. In learning to generate power and apply force it is important to examine ways to source and transmit power and the avenues through which it is delivered.

"To put the least amount of stress on your muscles, it is important to have as vertical an axis as possible while working at a massage table. Imagine that your spine is a plumb line that is attached from a hook above and weighted below. You are like a tree, with your feet like the roots, the torso like the trunk and your arms like the limbs. Stability and groundedness are at the feet and legs; direction of movement begins at the torso, and expression is through the arms and hands. By keeping the joints slightly bent and relaxed, the feet can step lightly and softly to produce a strong and fluid movement. Wherever the feet are pointed, the hips will move in that direction, and wherever the hips move, the arms and hands will follow. Feet are positioned squarely under the knees, hips and shoulders. Be aware of your field of movement. If your arms extend outward, be sure to maintain your solid base beneath."

June Lordi,
Massage Therapy Journal,
Summer 2003,
Vol. 42, No. 2, pg. 52

Sourcing and Transmitting Power

Power is sourced via *ground points* and transmitted by distributing weight, force and energy through *contact points*. By *ground points* we mean the very place from which power is generated; the place of origin, the starting point of an action or the root of a *wave*. These points are the stable points from which to originate and initiate power. By pushing into the *ground points*, therapists generate physical power, creating a *wave*, which moves through their entire *body* and is delivered to the client through the *contact points*.

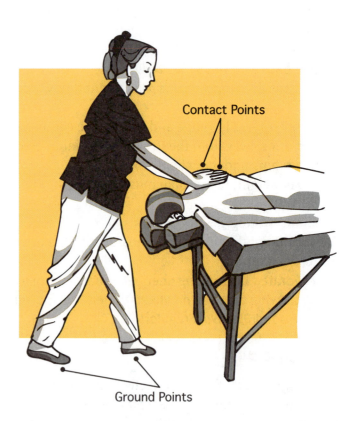

When standing: power is sourced through the feet (ground points) and delivered through the hands (contact points).

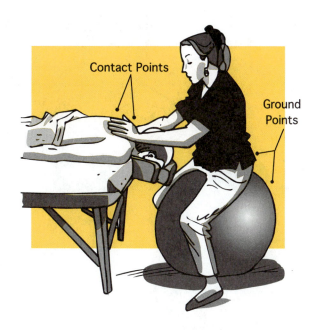

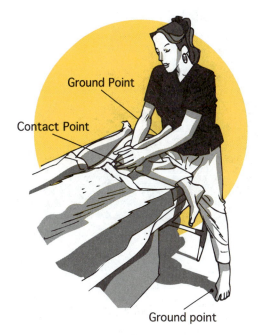

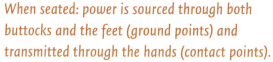

When seated: power is sourced through both buttocks and the feet (ground points) and transmitted through the hands (contact points).

When sitting table-side: power is sourced through the left foot and right buttock (ground points) and transmitted through the hands (contact points).

When standing next to the table, the feet will be the *ground points.* When seated on the side of the table, the *ground points* will be the foot on the floor and the buttock on the table. When seated on a stool, chair or ball, the *ground points* will be both buttocks and the feet. When working on the floor, the *ground points* might be the knees, feet, etc.

The *contact points* are the points of the *body*, such as the hands, feet, elbows, forearms, knees, etc., through which power is transmitted to the client's *body*. These *contact points* also receive information and responses back from the client. This creates the *feedback loop*, which forms the basis of the conversation that is *BodyWork*.

Trajectory or Path of Force

A *trajectory* is a path, projection or line of transmission. *Trajectories of force* are the passageways for transfer of power between *ground points* and *contact points*. These pathways can be vertical, horizontal, diagonal, circular, spiral and infinite combinations of shape, size and direction. A therapist, by visualizing pathways from him/herself to the client, can consciously send and receive power, energy and information.

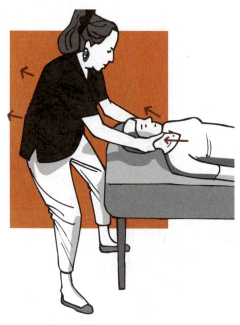

Leaning back and lifting creates a trajectory and path of force away from the trunk in a cranial and anterior direction.

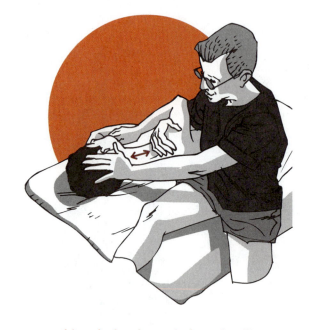

Pushing the head superiorly and pulling the shoulder inferiorly creates oppositional trajectories and paths of force.

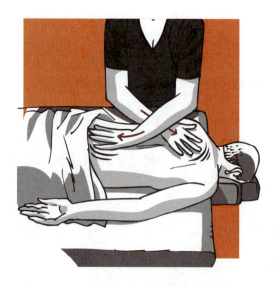

Moving simultaneously caudally and cranially creates multiple trajectories and paths of force.

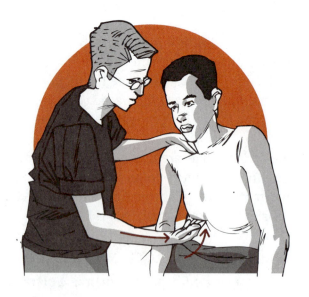

Pushing into the abdomen and up under the ribs creates a posterior and superior trajectory and path of force.

Therapists create a *trajectory of force* as they position themselves to come in at a particular angle, from a specific direction, with a measured amount of lean, push or pull. Intention may determine the location, the angle and direction of the *trajectory*. A practitioner may change the direction and angle of a *trajectory*, or combine multiple *trajectories*, in order to maintain the intention of an action/session. It is important for practitioners to position and mobilize themselves, consciously using *trajectories of force*, to transfer their power.

Experiential Exercise

1. **Face a wall**

2. **Place both hands on the wall at shoulder height**

3. **Lean into your hands and generate power from your shoulders, sending energy out into the wall**

4. **Observe the trajectories of force and how weight and energy travel in your body. Feel what you do with your body to generate your movements**

5. **Monitor your actions in response to the energy and pressure coming back from the wall**

6. **Repeat the above exercise generating power from your hips and then from your feet**

7. **Repeat again and change the angle of your lean**

8. **Notice how you function in each position. Look for similarities and differences**

Energy Exchange

Given that when we touch someone else we are touched back, one of the perks of *BodyWork* is the energy exchange. Good *body mechanics* leads to an unobstructed flow of energy that can be equally beneficial and enlivening for the therapist. In the giving is receiving, the *feedback loop* is continual, so it is not unusual for a practitioner to feel more vital and balanced after a session.

Work Surfaces

For the most part *BodyWork* is performed at a table. Some *modalities*, predominantly those from the East, are delivered on the floor. Others use chairs, cushions, mats, beds, balls, or specialized tables. While the actual physical delivery of *techniques* would be different depending on the type of surface that holds the *body*, the underlying principles of *body mechanics* are generally the same regarding posture, form and movement.

Whether you're standing, sitting or squatting you want to be as graceful, skillful and connected as possible. No matter what the work surface, it's important that you use yourself efficiently and comfortably (remember to employ the strategies and concepts discussed on page 26). Be aware of how you move through space and how you incorporate the elements of leverage and alignment in your work. Notice how you modify your posture and position. Pay attention as you source power from your ground points and deliver it in specific trajectories through your contact points. As you work, picture yourself being poised and powerful— a seamless flow of combinations of posture, balance, direction, locomotion, stillness, strength, intention and angle.

Table Height

If the work surface is a table, a critical factor in support of good *body mechanics* is the height. The type of work being done initially determines the table height. Lighter, more energy focused *modalities* are well served by using a higher table that allows for extended periods of light holding. Deeper work requires a lower table to keep *body* weight behind the hands so one uses less effort to achieve the desired effect. When using combinations of light and deep work it is beneficial for therapists to accommodate the lower height and support the periods of light holding by sitting on a stool or chair. This will bring them into a better relationship with the client's *body*.

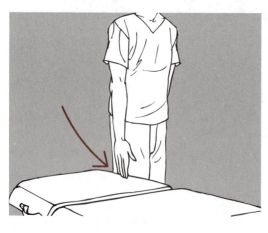

A good rule of thumb: measure to the tip of the longest finger when shoulders are relaxed and arm is hanging comfortably at one side.

Table height is also largely influenced by the structural proportion, strength and flexibility of the therapist. The ratio of a person's legs to trunk to arms may require setting the table a notch or two higher or lower than the "rule of thumb" identified at left. The strength and flexibility of therapists' legs affects how they can navigate around the table. If a therapist is not physically fit enough to accommodate the work needed for the *modality* utilized, it is important to do strength and/or flexibility training to develop optimal *body mechanics*.

A good rule of thumb when using deeper tissue or combined tissue/energy work is to set the top of the table at the level of the tip of the longest finger when the shoulders are relaxed and the arms are comfortably hanging at one's side. This measurement accommodates the depth of the "average" *body* and allows good leverage for deeper work. When massaging a bigger or a smaller person it might be necessary to lower or raise the table beyond this baseline setting. Some *modalities* (e.g., Rolfing and Connective Tissue Massage) suggest even lower height adjustments while others (e.g., Trager, Polarity and Kinergetics) recommend higher settings.

There are a number of points to consider when focusing on functional patterns. Using the following list of questions can spark an inner quest for self-awareness to support better use of a practitioner's whole being.

- **How am I "doing" what I'm "doing"?**

- **What does my "doing" feel like to me or my client?**

- **Is my "doing" getting the results I want?**

- **Can I feel when the client shifts as a result of my "doing"?**

- **What am I using/thinking/feeling as I do what I do?**

- **What in my body is moving/not moving?**

- **Where am I moving/bending/twisting/stabilizing from?**

- **What's happening in my spine?**

- **Where is the weight distributed in my feet?**

- **What's my posture in relation to my movements?**

- **How am I facing the table, the client's body or a specific body part?**

- **Am I connected to my inner core?**

Awareness and Adjustments

Body mechanics requires regular *proprioceptive* attention to one's *body* in relation to actions, intentions and client response. A self-*assessment* will reveal *facilitated pathways* of behavior that become ingrained over a lifetime. A *facilitated pathway* is a neural response pattern embedded in the nervous system by repetition associated with a learned activity. Repetition creates habits, which become the behavioral default. It takes conscious effort to override an existing pathway so the ideal is to embed the best possible patterns into the nervous system from the start. When we are conscious of what we are doing, we can personally shift the pathway toward optimal function.

It is beneficial for therapists to establish a system of self-awareness to keep tabs of their own *body* throughout a *BodyWork* session. Regular scanning during a session identifies the areas where it's possible to "lose" optimal patterns of movement. Once one becomes aware of inefficiently using a specific area or *body* part, it is important to make adjustments right away. Likewise, making a conscious note of what *is* working will lock optimal behavior into memory and create *facilitated pathways* in support of effective *body mechanics*.

One method promoting self-awareness involves creating a mental checklist or *mantra* to use during scanning. For example, "head, arms, hips and power source" or "shoulder down, hips forward, power from my feet." Using a list or *mantra* that emphasizes the areas to focus on will embed better patterns. It is a simple process to mentally repeat a list or *mantra* while passing the mind's eye through your *body*. Note how you feel, observe when an area is "off" and make the necessary adjustments right then and there.

Each and every action made by a practitioner is constantly modified depending on the *modality* and purpose, and the client's responses to initial and subsequent actions. It's an ongoing process that keeps one moving and adjusting and readjusting and redefining.

Sometimes practitioners will choose to get off balance and compromise some area of their own *body* in order to apply a *technique* in a "perfect" way to accomplish some exquisite move. Used sparingly, it can enable you to deliver to a particular intent. However, physical and energetic misalignment cannot become an ongoing standard of behavior. Constant torque, twist and strain, just might, and in all likelihood probably would, produce repetitive stress injuries that compromise form and function. Poor maintenance over time is abusive and can become a major threat to one's career. "Bad" *body mechanics* is professional suicide.

Learning *body mechanics* is a joint exploration for both student and teacher. It is a journey of discovery for "right" combinations of posture and movement. Finding and mastering the movement and form of one's own best *body mechanics* leads to BodyWork that is efficient, effective and empowering. Remember, good form not only varies from therapist to therapist, it changes even for the individual therapist, depending on the *modality* used, one's energy level, the table height or the client's size, shape, weight and condition.

So Why Use Good Body Mechanics?

Because good body mechanics will...

- **Provide longevity and stamina on a daily basis and for the life of a career**

- **Promote sensitivity and responsiveness to the client's condition/state**

- **Support the effective/precise application of intended skills**

- **Allow for greater subtlety and control in the delivery of skills**

- **Energize the practitioner**

- **Prevent strain and potential injury for both the practitioner and the client**

"Effective body use on the practitioner's part is a(n)...essential element...you generate resistance in your client if you muscle your way in, [and] your hands and shoulders will likely not serve you well for a long career. Fall into the tissue, and let it melt. The absolute minimum force to get the job done while maintaining maximum sensitivity to the many levels of the client's state...is our goal here."

Tom Myers,
Anatomists Corner,
Massage & BodyWork,
August/September 2004,
Vol. xix, No. 4, pg. 90

chapter **6**

Ergonomics

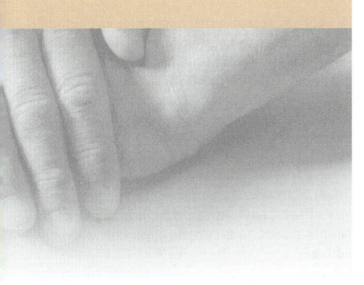

Ergonomics

Linda Riach

Once people dedicate themselves to a *BodyWork* career, and to building a practice, logical questions are, "How long can I do this? Is this a lifetime career?" The difference between a "no" and a "yes" answer often can be found in *ergonomics*.

What Is Ergonomics?

According to the Ergonomics Society of America, *ergonomics* is an approach that puts human needs and capabilities at the focus of designing products and work systems. The aim is to ensure that people and technology operate in harmony, so that there are fewer errors, repetitive strain injuries and work-related accidents, thereby promoting greater effectiveness. Fewer accidents and strains mean greater longevity and productivity, which contribute to a more robust livelihood and the ability to help more people.

BodyWork can be physically demanding and the wear and tear on a therapist's *body* can be debilitating. Injuries can occur in almost any area— from strained thumbs, fingers and hands, to hips, neck and lower back. Although the importance of proper *body mechanics* can be (and usually is) taught in schools, the truth is that the therapist is only half the equation. The other piece contributing to the longevity or brevity of a *BodyWork* career is the therapeutic equipment— tables, stools, chairs, mats and accessories. Realizing that the equipment is integral to the therapist's career, those who design with *ergonomics* in mind take the use of the apparatus *and* the therapist's *body mechanics* into account.

Underlying all *ergonomics* is careful analysis of human activity. The designer must understand all of the demands being made on the practitioner's hands, back, knees, hips, legs, etc., and the likely effects of supportive or unsupportive *body mechanics*. In *BodyWork*, *ergonomics* is demonstrated in a table's design through height, width and access-oriented features that allow close work in effective positions; stability, which maximizes the therapist's impact while minimizing movement; and material choice for health, strength and safety.

Another key ingredient is the understanding of how it all affects the work. Great *ergonomics* for the therapist doesn't mean much if the client isn't comfortable, safe, relaxed and receptive. The need to allow for human variability is critical because clients with a wide range of capabilities and limitations present for treatment. Regarding *BodyWork* tables, *ergonomics* is demonstrated through features such as adjustable height (electronic or manual), including extra-low range (e.g., for ease of getting on and off); foam softness (e.g., for client comfort); tilt function (e.g., for sinus and cardiac issues); and environmentally friendly fabric composition (e.g., to minimize allergy-related sensitivities). Chairs, stools, bolsters and other equipment can also be designed with these principles in mind.

Ergonomically designed equipment also takes into consideration the *modality* and functionality of the individual practitioner. Not all equipment can be designed to do all jobs ergonomically. An intimate knowledge of *body mechanics* for a specific type of work is central to choosing the right equipment. For example, the demands of structural integration are going to be different from those of energy work. Structural integration practices, such as Rolfing, are best supported by a table that is low, for leverage; strong, to support compressive *techniques*; and wide, to provide space for the therapist to be on the table too. On the other hand, energy practitioners are often seated and need to move freely around a table without cables or understructures being in the way.

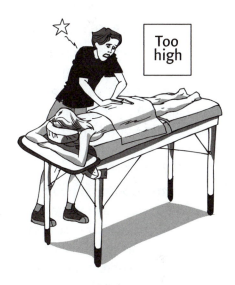

Too high

Ergonomics Humanizes Technology

The commitment to "human-centered design" has an essential "humanizing" effect on the rapid developments in technology that are influencing our lives. If a company designs a product that works to the benefit of the practitioner and the client, it is a win/win scenario allowing both parties to derive maximum value and minimum wear and tear. When a table or tool is ergonomically smart it essentially disappears as it is seamlessly incorporated into the treatment, becoming a natural extension of the practitioner/client relationship. The impact is simple, yet profound. Practitioners who minimize or eliminate the wear and tear on their own *body* will have a longer, more fulfilling career.

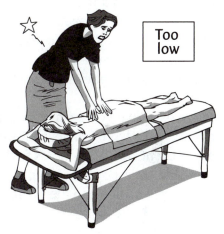

Too low

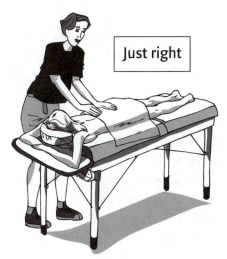

Just right

What to Look for (and Avoid) in Table Enhancements

Table innovations are rapidly developing and can be confusing to the therapist. On the positive side, there are qualities in many tables that enhance and support various *modalities*. There are also several new, seemingly ergonomic-friendly innovations on the market that should be approached with a bit of caution and regard. Though well-meaning, some table features can actually cause problems, rather than prevent them.

PADDING

Appropriate padding supports both the client and the therapist, allowing clients the comfort they need and giving way for the therapists' hands when necessary. Padding that doesn't "relax" out of the way to allow for easy access under the client's *body* can inhibit treatment and wear down a practitioner's hands. The key here is the resilience or responsiveness of the padding. Does it provide support, filling in the body's contours while also being pliable? There is now a generation of high-quality foams that demonstrate these "smart" qualities, seeming to know what the client wants and needs. Are men and women both comfortable and well-supported when lying prone? Or is breast pain a serious concern? Remember, too, softer is not always better. Some *modalities*, like Shiatsu, are more effective with firmer, less-giving padding because firmness supports the *localized* pressure inherent in the treatment. Softer padding would diffuse the impact.

A word of warning on the heat-responsive foams like those used in mattresses. The very qualities that make the high-tech foam sleep-inducing can jeopardize the therapist and cause discomfort for the client. The foam molds to the client's body and stays in that shape because it is designed to be slow to respond to changes (the characteristic is called "memory"). So, in short, the client is in a new position and the foam isn't, or at least not for a while. This foam is designed to compress. That's fine on a bed, but there are only a few inches of foam on a *BodyWork* table. It often compresses right down to the plywood at the base of the table top. When it compresses completely, two things happen: 1) the client perceives the table as "hard" and 2) the therapists' hands, wrists and knuckles bear tremendous weight as they are pressed into the table frame. To further exacerbate the scenario, a portable table constructed with the new foam is actually very heavy and not very portable at all.

ACCESS ENDS

Access ends allow the therapist greater comfort when sitting. They provide unobstructed leg room which permits closer contact with the client and supports efficient *body mechanics*. Therapists can easily test an access end design to see if it is right for them by adjusting their stool/chair/ball and table height so that their forearms can rest comfortably on the table. If so, and their knees slide easily under the table as well, it's a good fit. If they have to raise the table to get their knees underneath, their shoulders will also rise, causing neck and back strain.

ARM RESTS

An arm rest is an extension off the end of a table which hangs below the face cradle to support the client's arms in a forward position while lying prone. Well-designed arm rests relax the clients' shoulder girdle, allowing them to comfortably lie prone for extended periods. Clients with restricted shoulder *mobility* may need an arm rest to comfortably lie prone.

SHAPED TABLES

Tables that are shaped on the sides allow practitioners to get closer to clients. This provides better access to the client's lower torso with less twisting, reaching and stretching for the practitioner.

ESSENTIAL LIFTS

For those therapists in a permanent office setting, nonportable tables with mechanical or electrical lift mechanisms can be ideal. This beneficial table innovation supports practitioners in a myriad of unprecedented ways:

- It is adjustable to any height within its range, which optimizes the practitioners' *body mechanics* for any size client and any *modality*
- It lowers and raises with minimal effort, saving practitioners' bodies for their practice
- It allows the practitioner to be more responsive to the issues clients present as it seamlessly supports a variety of *modalities* within any session without inconveniencing the client or practitioner
- It accommodates clients who have difficulty getting on and off the table, thus reducing the strain on both the practitioner and the client

Many practitioners find that the regular use of a lift table alleviates a significant portion of the *body* fatigue they often experience at the end of the day.

"Most therapists use a work stool to sit on while performing certain techniques. A cushioned stool with good rolling wheels is the most efficient type of seating while you work. Another comfortable substitute for a good stool is to work while sitting on a large exercise ball."

Ben Benjamin,
Massage Therapy Journal,
Spring 2004,
Vol. 43, No. 1, pg. 33

"Ergonomics is the evaluation of how well the environments you work and live in support what you do there.... Using our bodies in the most relaxed and efficient manner—both at work and in life—helps us to avoid fatigue, overuse injury and eventual burnout. The work and living environments that we create either support our health or diminish it.... I learned how to construct my environment so that it did not deplete energy, but rather added to my productivity."

Ben Benjamin,
Massage Therapy Journal,
Spring 2004,
Vol. 43, No. 1, pg. 30

Other Considerations

EQUIPMENT TRANSPORT

Carrying a *massage* chair or table can be a tiring, possibly injurious challenge. Carrying aids reduce or eliminate the strain of transporting equipment across parking lots and down long hallways. This helps to keep the practitioner fresh from client to client. Aids include table carts, luggage wheelies and specialized bags. Table carts may be the easiest to use as they are designed specifically for this purpose. When choosing a lug-

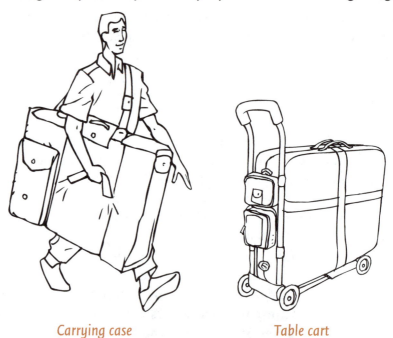

Carrying case   Table cart

gage wheelie, select one with a handle that extends above the table when it's on its end and with wheels sturdy enough to keep the whole thing stable while moving. Carrying cases, as an alternative, have the advantage of spreading the weight between the shoulder and the opposite hip while allowing free use of hands to open doors, etc. (They also protect the table surface from damage.)

CUSHIONS, BOLSTERS AND RECESSES

No two people are alike. Distances between clients' breasts and chin, differences between breast shapes and sizes or relationships of any *body* parts vary by individual. Adjustable cushions, bolsters, contoured cushion systems and tables with variable positioning can do wonders to create comfort because they are infinitely adaptable and can be "customized" to fit each client. It is important to note that built-in recesses (or holes), which are static and aren't adjustable to meet every *body*, can force the client into an uncomfortable position. Practitioners also need to be aware of the potential issues regarding pregnancy recesses. Although it seems to make sense to accommodate a pregnant woman's growing abdomen, allowing too much belly to hang through the recess may add unwarranted stress on already stretched and taxed ligaments, blood vessels and muscles.

The role of *ergonomics* is as critical an ingredient in a *BodyWork* career as knowledge, *skill* and passion for the work. No other single factor contributes more profoundly to the longevity and effectiveness of one's practice. When buying equipment, it is important to know that those who designed it have done so with true *ergonomics* in mind— taking its principles *and* the therapist's *body mechanics* into account. Your body and your clients will thank you.

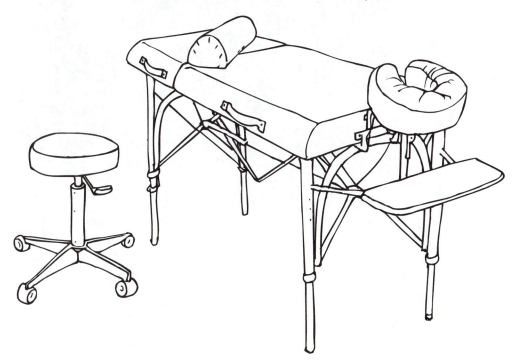

Table with arm rest, face cradle, bolster, access ends and a stool

part

II

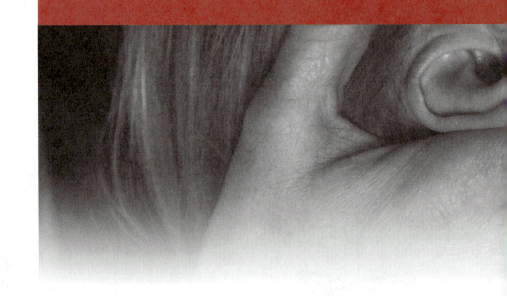

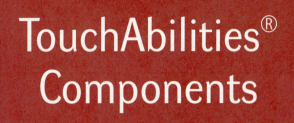

TouchAbilities®
Components

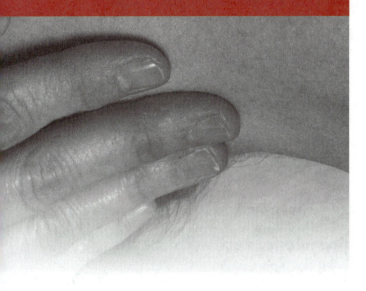

Flash Warning!

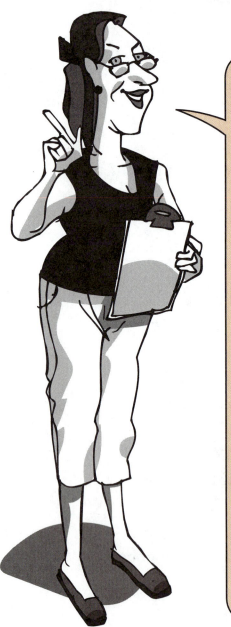

The TouchAbilities® model is an arbitrary reduction of a unified whole. It is divided for instructional purposes only... a simplified organization of ideas and skills to get you to the realm beyond division.

A *body* is a dynamic integrated, *multidimensional* field.

The tangible/physical world of anatomy and physiology is activated by the intangible energetic aspects of invisible fields, lines, flows, channels and connections and vice versa.

TouchAbilities® Skill Chart

Breathing Component

tracking
directing
pacing

Cognitive Component

visualizing
inquiring
intending
focusing
transmitting

Energetic Component

sensing
intuiting
balancing

Compression Component

pressing/pushing
squeezing/pinching
twisting/wringing

Expansion Component

pulling
lifting
rolling

Kinetic Component

holding/supporting
mobilizing
letting go/dropping
stabilizing

Oscillation Component

vibrating
shaking
striking

Gliding Component

sliding/planing
rubbing

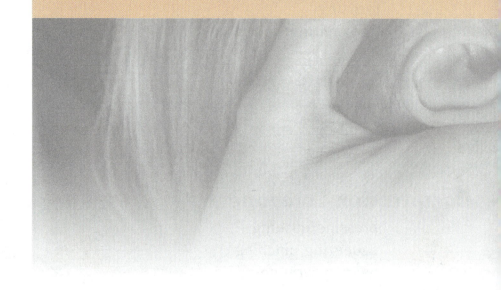

chapter **7**

Breathing Component

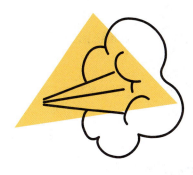

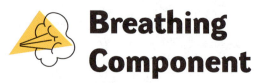

Breathing Component

Introduction

Breath is life, the link between our corporal *body* and our spirit essence. It animates our physical being. It provides the fuel for every vital function.

It is the *carrier wave* for aliveness, movement and flow. It is an involuntary process that allows for some voluntary control. Each and every moment, with or without our awareness, the *body* meets the physical demands of all its systems. We can consciously override these autonomic patterns to influence speed, power, depth, *rhythm*, location, duration of breath, and the muscular activity involved in breathing.

Respiration drives an essential exchange of nutrient and waste gases through the lungs. Inhalation into the lungs brings nutrient gases to the blood and heart. The heart propels these gases via the blood to every cell in the *body*. Inversely, metabolic waste gases are carried through the blood to the heart and lungs and expelled through exhalation. (This is a highly simplified description of the process. Refer to a physiology text for more specific details.)

We take thousands of breaths each day. The mechanics of breathing involve the diaphragm, muscles of the ribs and neck and various other muscles, tissues and organs. The movement of these structures during breathing creates *waves* that impact every system of the *body*. This impact translates to pulsation, excitation, movement, vitality, *motility* and connection.

The three primary skills that can be applied when using the breath as a therapeutic tool are:

TRACKING— taking notice of the pattern of inhalation and exhalation

DIRECTING— consciously and intentionally influencing the flow of inhalation and exhalation

PACING— coordinating the actions and/or breath of the therapist with the breath *wave* of the client (work follows breath *wave*)

"Massage therapy is an excellent opportunity to focus and move your own body as you are helping your client. Every time we inhale, we are gathering strength for the next movement. Each exhale effectively executes that movement with efficiency and gracefulness. The mind must always be focused on its intention, whether it is the bodyworker delivering the massage, the athlete playing his or her sport or the laborer at work."

June Lordi,
Massage Therapy Journal,
Summer 2003,
Vol. 42, No. 2, pg. 51

Tracking: taking notice of the pattern of inhalation and exhalation

SYNONYMS: studying, exploring, scanning, scrutinizing, watching, observing

INTENTIONS
- To note breathing cycle and pattern (regularity/irregularity)
- To identify how breath is initiated and expressed (chest/abdomen; mouth/nose)
- To note depth and breadth of cycle (shallow/deep; full/restricted)
- To monitor the body's response to application of techniques

This is not a definitive list of intentions. It is a sampling of possibilities designed to stimulate your learning. As you discover other options, add them to the list.

TRACKING is taking notice of the pattern of inhalation and exhalation- the breath *wave*. It means to study, explore, scan and scrutinize the way breath moves through the *body*. Ideally, the passage of air is animated and expressed in a free and easy respiratory cycle. Optimal breathing requires a *body* that is flexible, elastic, responsive and vital. By following the breath through the nose and mouth, neck and throat, chest, back and belly, down to the pelvis, both the practitioner and the client can note its path, which areas expand first, which ones follow, and which ones are restricted. Locations where inconsistencies are noted can indicate areas of holding on any level—physical, emotional, mental and/or spiritual. **TRACKING** depth, breadth, *rhythm*, effort, restrictions and/or irregularities and the still point between inhalation and exhalation enables the therapist to identify a focus and purpose for therapeutic applications. Breathing patterns often change as other shifts occur in the *body*. **TRACKING** the breath can be used throughout a session to check a person's response to various *techniques* and other stimuli.

PRACTITIONER'S ACTIONS - TRACKING

Employ your senses of touch, sight, smell and hearing to notice the client's pattern of inhalation and exhalation.

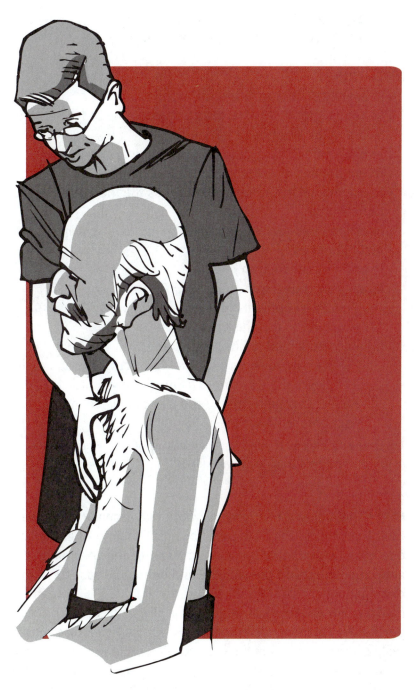

Directing: consciously and intentionally influencing the flow of inhalation and exhalation

SYNONYMS: guiding, leading, engaging, regulating, affecting, adapting, managing, training, controlling, inviting, encouraging

INTENTIONS
- To expand or compress internal structures
- To access specific *body* areas from within the *body* itself (using compressive and expansive forces of the breathing mechanism)
- To oxygenate the *body* and vitalize life-force energy
- To explore and affect tension
- To use the outside force of air *waves* as the therapist projects his/her own breath at the client's *body*
- To use focused awareness on the breath as a *technique* for centering, autosuggestion, meditation, etc.
- To assist or enhance an intention
- To alter breathing patterns to:
    - establish optimal breathing patterns
    - connect to the energy of the universe
    - access sacred realms
    - shift consciousness and *brainwave* activity (beta, alpha, theta, delta)
    - influence the wave form using diaphragmatic breathing
    - effect change using the still point between in/out breath
    - support self-awareness

This is not a definitive list of intentions. It is a sampling of possibilities designed to stimulate your learning. As you discover other options, add them to the list.

DIRECTING is used to consciously and intentionally influence the flow of inhalation and exhalation. This process can be initiated by the client and/or guided by the therapist. Engaging, inviting, encouraging, leading, regulating, managing and controlling the breath *wave* produces numerous and varied effects on the tangible and intangible aspects of the *body*. On a core level, it supports oxygenation, and vitalizes life force energy. **DIRECTED** breathing can be instrumental in releasing held tension and stress throughout the *body* and correcting respiratory pattern distortions. It supports self-awareness, shifts consciousness and *brainwave* activity and connects a person to sacred realms and the energy of the universe. The breath can be used to assist or enhance an intention or as a force for change. It is a dynamic way to use the compressive and expansive forces of the breathing mechanism within the *body* itself, to access and affect internal structures.

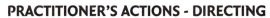

PRACTITIONER'S ACTIONS - DIRECTING

Use your own breath, physical contact and/or verbal communication to influence the client's breathing cycle.

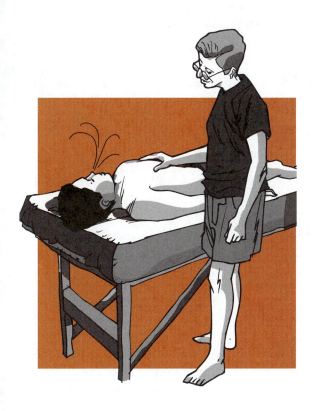

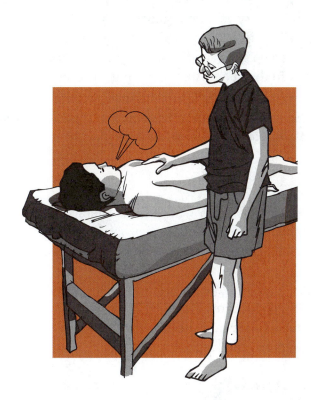

Pacing: coordinating the actions and/or breath of the therapist with the breath wave of the client (work follows breath wave)

SYNONYMS: following, entraining, aligning, synchronizing, attuning, corresponding, resonating, coordinating, harmonizing, correlating, keeping time with, acting in unison, coinciding, matching

INTENTIONS
- To come into harmony or resonance with client
- To gain insight into client's *state*
- To direct client's awareness of his/her own breath
- To carry an intention or information
- To soften the intensity of *body* sensations and/or the treatment application
- To heighten and/or amplify effect of the treatment
- To direct a shift in breathing patterns
- To access an optimal moment or position in the breathing cycle for effective intervention

This is not a definitive list of intentions. It is a sampling of possibilities designed to stimulate your learning. As you discover other options, add them to the list.

PACING is a *skill* whereby the therapist coordinates his/her breath with that of the client. By matching inhalations and exhalations, the practitioner entrains to, follows and uses the client's breath *wave* or creates and exaggerates his/her own breath *wave* to influence the client.

By matching breath patterns, a therapist can come into harmony and resonance with a client. This connection allows the therapist to "step into the client's being" to gain insight into his or her *state*. This establishes a relationship on the most primal level and sets a baseline from which a therapist can respond.

PACED breathing can carry an intention, or information anywhere on/in the *body*. It can support the client to become aware of his/her own breath. It can soften the intensity of, or heighten and amplify the effects of a particular treatment application. It can also be used with **DIRECTED** breathing to support a shift in breath pattern.

PRACTITIONER'S ACTIONS - PACING

Adjust your breathing cycle and/or other *BodyWork* applications to match the client's breathing cycle.

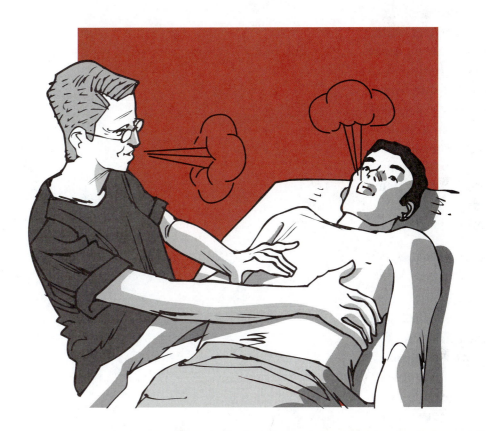

"Breathing is the one function of the body which is directly responsive to both our voluntary and autonomic nervous systems, and it is a key bridge between the conscious and unconscious. The breath is a primary source of our energy and vibration.... The response of the breath pattern is a direct signal of the energy shifts in the body."

Fritz Frederick Smith, MD,
Inner Bridges, 1986

"Entrainment... involves the ability of the more powerful rhythmic vibrations of one object to change the less powerful vibrations of another object and cause them to synchronize their rhythms with the first object."

Jonathan Goldman, Healing Sounds, 1996

"A three-dimensional experience of pulsating 'volume' is created when we breathe fully and touch. Touch with breath conveys to our clients life itself, vitality, spirit, and rhythm. The breath, not our hands, is the primary energy source for our work and life."

David Lauterstein, Massage Therapy Journal, Spring/Summer 1997, Vol.36, No.2, pg.119

Experientials

Breathing Component

These exploratory activities are designed to provide a direct experience of the *skills* introduced in this chapter. They are combined and integrated with other *skills* that would naturally occur in an actual *BodyWork* practice. Try them out and observe the results. As you gain proficiency and understand the effects, be inspired to create your own applications.

1. As a person breathes, watch the rise and fall of his ribs.

2. Tell a client to inhale through her nostrils and exhale through her mouth, then have her reverse this and inhale through her mouth and out through her nostrils.

3. Guide a client to breathe into your hands as you place them on different parts of his body (rib cage, feet, trigger point, chakra, reflex point).

4. Match your breathing rhythm with that of your client.

5. Accentuate the sound of your breath so the client can hear you; note if she follows your lead.

6. Have a client inhale, while focusing on a tender point; then, exhale as you visualize the point releasing.

7. Observe a client's breath as you compress and broaden her quadriceps.

8. Direct a client to inhale to a count of 5 and exhale to a count of 8.

9. Note when a client takes in a spontaneous deep breath and releases with a sigh.

10. Release your pressure as a client inhales.

Modalities Using Breathing Component Skills

Breathing Component *skills* can be incorporated into any therapeutic relationship and combined with any *modality*. However, there are *modalities* that feature these *skills* as an integral part of their system.

Some examples are:
Bhakti Energy Work™*
Chi Kung
Feldenkrais Method™*
Holotropic Breathwork
Inside-Out Paradigm*
Meditation
Mother Massage®*
Multi-Dimensional Movement
  Arts (MDMA)®*
Natural Childbirth
NMT*
Past-Life Regression
Pranayama Yoga
Rebirthing
Structural Integration
Tai Chi
Toning
Trager® Approach
Waterdance
Yamuna® Body Logic*
Yamuna® Body Rolling*

*See Linking TouchAbilities®
to Modalities, chapter 23.

chapter **8**

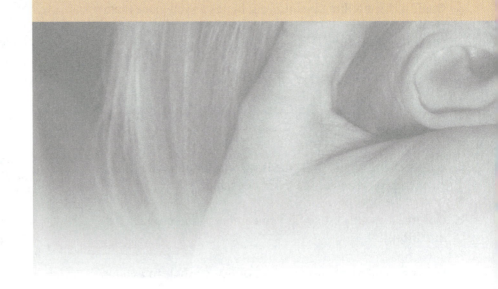

Cognitive Component

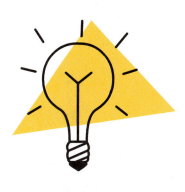

"A good practitioner is helping the client to learn how to 'control the controls' of our essentially conservative yet radically open-ended sensorimotor creativity.... New images suggest new kinds of movement and new possible strategies... [which] challenge the parameters of previous beliefs... [and] can alter not only the specific instances in which a specific resistance is encountered, but a whole world view that creates resistance per se.... It is clear that bodywork must reach the mind in order to effect genuine and lasting changes of this kind."

Dean Juhan,
Massage Magazine,
March/April 1995,
No.54, pg. 63

Cognitive Component

Introduction

COGNITIVE *skills* can greatly enhance and magnify the impact of all physical manipulations. These *skills* arise from the mind, which is distinct from the brain. The brain is a physical structure located in the *body*, and the mind is intangible and beyond the limits of the physical construct.

The world is experienced through images that appear on our mental screen. *Thoughtwaves* and mental images carry ideas, information and intentions. Humans can communicate and interact with all living forms using these *waves* and images to manipulate and impact reality. Thoughts, ideas, prayers, dreams, etc., are *nonlocal* and can be used to cause effects over distance and time.

INQUIRING, INTENDING, VISUALIZING, FOCUSING and **TRANSMITTING** are the **Cognitive** tools for *assessment*, enhancement, modification and change. Applied alone, or in combination with touch, they can have a profound effect on the way a person experiences him/herself in the universe.

VISUALIZING— picturing in one's mind; seeing a mental image of something

INQUIRING— questing for truth, knowledge or information; verbal and nonverbal asking

INTENDING— consciously establishing a purpose or plan; directing energy toward a goal

FOCUSING— concentrating awareness on a selected point of attention

TRANSMITTING— consciously conveying or sending out a signal, i.e., thought, image, feeling, idea, intention, color, sound, etc.

"Our language for describing physical sensation lends itself to somatic imaging. We are accustomed to using metaphors to describe our physical condition. A 'stabbing' pain, a 'wrenched' neck, a 'churned up' stomach, a 'burning' sensation, a 'shooting' pain, a 'pins and needle' sensation, a 'tight' muscle are examples of the images embedded within commonly used phrases."

Clyde Ford,
Where Healing Waters Meet, 1989

Visualizing: picturing in one's mind; seeing a mental image of something

SYNONYMS: picturing, visioning, imagining, conjuring up, calling up, creating, viewing, fantasizing, contemplating, thinking of, conceiving

INTENTIONS
- To support self-discovery, healing, relaxation, problem solving, insight
- To envision possibilities of an idea or opportunity (an artist sees a beautiful sculpture in a piece of wood before creating it by hand)
- To work out details of a plan before manifesting it (an entrepreneur imagines the store filled with stock before renting the building and opening the doors for business)
- To improve performance (an athlete sees him/herself running in perfect form before entering the race)
- To promote shifts in the *body* (a person slows down his/her breathing by imagining being in a relaxed situation)
- To change cellular structure (a cancer patient holds an image of a vacuum cleaning up the tumor)
- To heal a condition (a person with a heart ailment images a healthy heart muscle)
- To achieve a desired goal (a person on a diet can see him/herself at an optimal weight)

This is not a definitive list of intentions. It is a sampling of possibilities designed to stimulate your learning. As you discover other options, add them to the list.

VISUALIZING is creating a picture in one's mind. A person can conceive an idea, develop a vision, imagine a goal or conjure up a mental image. This *skill* can assist in manifesting a dream or bringing a concept into concrete reality as when an artist sees the finished sculpture in the raw piece of marble or when an entrepreneur sees a store filled with stock before renting the space.

Envisioning possibilities allows a person to more easily recognize opportunities as they appear. **VISUALIZING** allows the therapist, the client or both to use a mentally held image for self-discovery, healing, relaxation, problem solving, pain management, and behavioral and functional modification. It promotes shifts in the *body* as when a person slows down his/her breathing by imagining him/herself in a relaxed situation. It can cause change on a cellular level as when a cancer patient holds an image of a vacuum consuming the tumor. It can assist in healing a condition as when a person with a heart ailment holds an image of a healthy heart muscle. **VISUALIZING** during a *BodyWork* session can affect releasing a trigger point, lengthening a muscle, opening an energy pathway, etc.

PRACTITIONER'S ACTIONS - VISUALIZING
Hold a mental image in your own mind and/or have the client do the same.

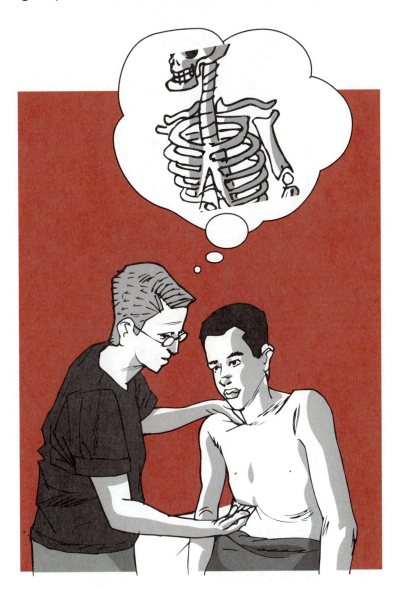

Holding a mental image to facilitate change

Three examples of VISUALIZING applications are:

Visualization, imagery for self-healing: The use of mental imagery to create changes in the *body*— cellularly, molecularly, energetically. The *body* continuously replaces cells. With conscious thought we may be able to influence the transferable information.

Creative Imagery: the ability to picture an idea before bringing it into physical reality

Guided Imagery:

    Externally generated— A script, spoken by a guide, designed to direct an inner mental journey

    Internally generated— Somatic Imaging: Imagery identified by the client and directed by the therapist. Process: Ask the client to describe an image (shape, size, color, texture, density, sensation, emotion, etc.) related to tension, pain, a specific point or a general area of the *body*. Then, direct a shift in this image to release or dissipate the focus area or reconnect the client to a greater awareness of his/her *body*.

"All bodywork is essentially a conversation between two intelligent systems. That conversation— especially when it is nonverbal— takes place in the language of relationship.... We do not 'fix' people, no matter how good we get; we inform their bodies, and they organize themselves into 'better.'"

Tom Myers,
Massage Magazine,
May/June 2000, pg.23

"Guided Imagery: n (noun)
1: deliberate, directed day dreaming; a purposeful use of the imagination that automatically alters consciousness.
2: evocative, multi-sensory meditation that causes deep shifts in body, psyche and spirit.
3: words, images & music that mobilize neurophysiology and biochemistry, producing a healing wave that surges through your body, soothing and nurturing every cell from top to bottom."

Belleruth Naparstek, www.conferenceworks.com, 2005

Inquiring: questing for truth, knowledge or information; verbal and nonverbal asking

SYNONYMS: examining, questioning, interviewing, interrogating, asking, probing, scrutinizing, analyzing, checking, testing, studying, investigating, searching, seeking, checking up, scoping out

INTENTIONS
- To express an idea/understanding
- To identify qualities and boundaries of physical and energetic fields (physical, emotional, mental and spiritual)
- To establish and maintain a line of communication between client and therapist
- To gather client information
- To monitor the client's experience
- To monitor the therapist's experience
- To establish and refine an intention for a session or course of treatment

This is not a definitive list of intentions. It is a sampling of possibilities designed to stimulate your learning. As you discover other options, add them to the list.

INQUIRING encompasses the quest for truth, knowledge and information. It is the verbal and nonverbal act of asking. Examine, interrogate, probe, scrutinize, analyze, test, study, investigate, search, seek and check-out exemplify this concept. To "bring a question to the table" in a *BodyWork* session is to be open to "what is so" in the moment. This includes a therapist interviewing a client to gather information and to set an INTENTION for the session. How do you feel? What would you like to accomplish today? Is there a specific area you want to focus on?

Inquiry assists in identifying qualities and boundaries of physical and energetic *fields*. What is the pliability of this tissue? How does this move and stretch? What's attached to the part/s being moved? How far can this joint be mobilized? Did you feel the energy expand through this part?

A therapist and/or client can "hold a question" as an underlying impetus for observing, assessing and responding to what is taking place. The therapist might think: What area or parts are not moving that should? What can be freer, lighter, easier? As this lets go, where else can I take it? This is not releasing, what else can I try? The client might hold the question: Where am I stuck? How can I let go? What does this mean to me?

This powerful, interactive tool can be used throughout a session to establish and maintain a line of communication for discovery and feedback. How is the pressure of my contact? Are you aware of this restriction? Tell me how you feel now? Did you notice that release?

PRACTITIONER'S ACTIONS - INQUIRING

Use your thought mechanisms and/or verbal skills to seek an answer to a query and/or have the client do the same.

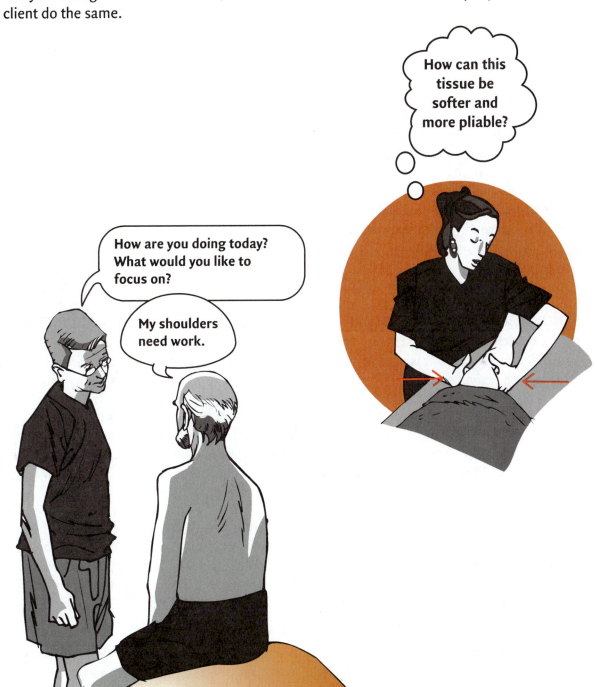

Intending: consciously establishing a purpose or plan; directing energy toward a goal

Synonyms: approaching, strategizing, designing, aiming, setting one's sights on, planning, having in mind, predetermining

INTENTIONS
- To establish a purpose for action
- To design a course of action
- To make firm that which is imagined
- To establish a measure for progress
- To facilitate change
- To serve the client's highest good
- To promote health, balance and *homeostasis*
- To work toward any other pertinent outcome

This is not a definitive list of intentions. It is a sampling of possibilities designed to stimulate your learning. As you discover other options, add them to the list.

INTENDING gives impetus to create and provides a purpose for action. It is an essential and integral part of a conscious *BodyWork* session. **INTENDING** establishes a purpose or plan; it directs effort toward a determined goal. It is used to strategize, design, aim, set one's sights on, have in mind or predetermine a desired outcome. This goal can be vocalized, written or held as a thought in the mind.

INTENTIONS define the nature of the client/practitioner relationship. They can be for the moment, the session or the course of treatment. They can be *localized* to a specific point of focus or can be more generalized involving an area or an entire *field*. They can be singular or multiple and can change moment to moment. Flexibility is a key to effective outcomes. It is essential in responding to the new influences that are always stimulating change and shifting the current *state* of things.

Setting a goal provides an ideal by which to measure client progress. During a session, the therapist can observe the current *state* of the client and compare this with the **INTENDED** outcome. For example, if an **INTENTION** is to expand the range of motion (ROM) of a joint, the therapist will occasionally check the *mobility* of that joint to see if the work is effective and when the goal is reached. Using **INTENTION** in this way will assist in knowing when and how to modify the application or course of action, or when a session is complete.

The benefits are intensified when an **INTENTION** is co-created by both therapist and client, and established and directed toward the highest good for all concerned. This *skill* empowers the work and facilitates the process toward balance, *homeostasis* and health on physical, emotional, mental and spiritual levels.

PRACTITIONER'S ACTIONS - INTENDING
Use your mind to consciously create a plan or purpose and/or have the client do the same.

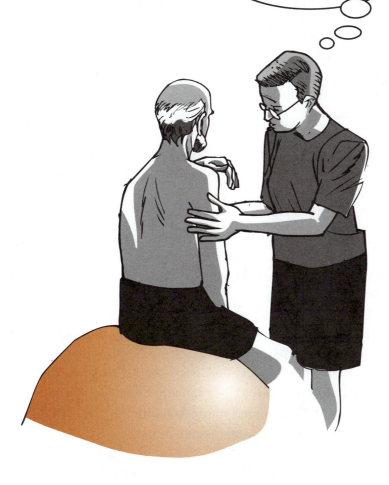

Focusing: concentrating awareness on a selected point of attention

SYNONYMS: directing attention, centering, emphasizing, distinguishing, concentrating, highlighting, lasering

INTENTIONS
- To integrate specific area/s with the whole
- To dissipate tension or pain in an area
- To identify mental or emotional aspects of sensations experienced in an area
- To direct an image of health or an *affirmation* for change regarding a specific area
- To establish conscious awareness of tension and holding patterns
- To achieve relaxation (physical, emotional, mental, spiritual)
- To bring energy to an area of focus

This is not a definitive list of intentions. It is a sampling of possibilities designed to stimulate your learning. As you discover other options, add them to the list.

FOCUSING concentrates awareness on a selected point of attention. It delineates and specifies a site to which we can deliver ideas, information and INTENTIONS. It is the act of taking aim at a target.

FOCUSING is used to *localize* physical manipulations, to dissipate tension or pain and/or to integrate a part to the whole. It is the act of placing attention onto any sensation, idea or location such as a trigger point, a prior experience or a *body* process. This is helpful when TRANSMITTING an image of health or an *affirmation* for change.

The act of **FOCUSING** allows one to center on, emphasize, distinguish, highlight and bring consciousness and awareness to sensations experienced in a particular area. Then, *thoughtwaves* and mental images can be "lasered" to that specific location. For example, when treating a tight muscle, the therapist can **FOCUS** his/her touch to that location and direct a client's attention to the exact point of discomfort. The client is then guided to breathe into that area, **FOCUS** on it during the in-breath and dissipate the sensation during the out-breath.

Progressive Relaxation is an example of **FOCUSING** where a client is guided through his/her *body* and led to sequentially contract and release specific muscles (see page 73).

PRACTITIONER'S ACTIONS - FOCUSING

Use and aim your conscious awareness at a target and/or have the client do the same.

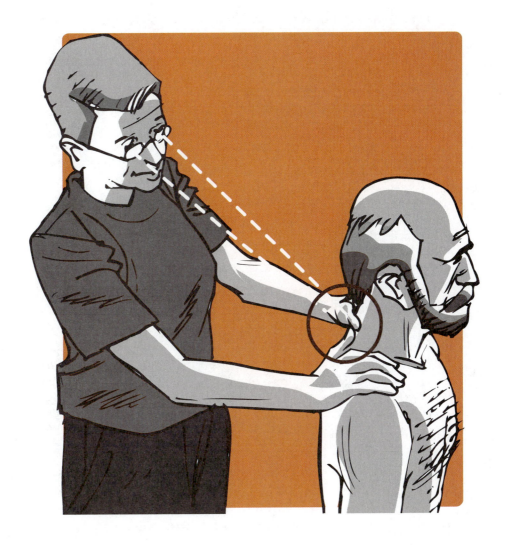

Experiential Exercise– Progressive Relaxation

1. Lie down on a flat surface and get into a comfortable open position with your legs slightly apart and your arms and hands by your sides.
2. Take several deep breaths and with each exhale sink into the flat surface.
3. Notice how you feel as you breathe rhythmically and gently.
4. Now take a big inhale and contract all the muscles in your feet.
5. On the exhale release those contracted muscles in your feet; envision your feet lengthening and releasing.
6. Take another big inhale and contract your calf muscles; intensify the tightness there.
7. On the exhale release your contracted calf muscles. Watch as the tension dissipates and your calves soften and elongate.
8. On the next inhale contract your quadriceps, the big muscles on the top of your thigh.
9. On your exhale release the quadriceps. Feel yourself melting and becoming lighter; notice how the back of your thigh and the rest of your legs feel.
10. Inhale and contract your buttocks muscles, your gluteals.
11. Release the gluteals as you exhale. Notice how your lower back relates to the surface beneath you.
12. Now as you inhale contract and squeeze your shoulder blades together.
13. As you exhale release your shoulder blades and feel the rhomboids relax, your shoulders open and your chest expand.
14. On this next inhale crunch up your neck and upper back muscles. Squeeze them tightly.
15. On the exhale release the neck and upper back muscles. Feel yourself sink into the surface as the bones of your spine separate and your neck elongates.
16. Now inhale and scrunch up all your facial muscles and clench your jaw.
17. Release those facial and jaw muscles on the exhale and let your face go limp. Feel your cheeks, jaw and forehead open and expand.
18. Now simultaneously contract and tighten every muscle in your body.
19. Hold this position for a few breaths and on an exhale let it all go.
20. Focus again on your breathing. Allow it to become slow, deep and gentle.
21. Close your eyes and rest.

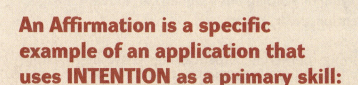

An Affirmation is a specific example of an application that uses INTENTION as a primary skill:

It is a strong, constructive, positive statement made to help realize goals. To affirm is to make an assertion or declaration, as if already true, about something that one desires to actualize. For example: "I am a creative and effective mother"; "I am a gentle spirit and a powerful energy source"; "I live in a state of grace: grounded, relaxed, aware, centered and energized."

"There are many practical applications of the principle that what we affirm and program into the unconscious belief system we tend in subtle ways to bring about. When we establish and affirm an intention or a goal, imagining that it is already so, the unconscious mind is programmed to achieve that goal even in ways which the conscious part of the mind does not plan or understand."

Willis Harman,
Global Mind Change, 1998

"...positive imagery activates the nervous system, sends neurohormones through the bloodstream and triggers healing activity"

Belleruth Naparstek,
"Intuition, Imagery & Healing"
seminar brochure, 2000.

Transmitting: consciously conveying or sending out a signal, i.e., thought, image, feeling, idea, intention, color, sound, etc.

SYNONYMS: communicating, transferring, delivering, broadcasting, conveying, passing on, disseminating, radiating, echoing, sending, diffusing

INTENTIONS
- To highlight the current state of a system (send out a signal that bounces back with information, perceived through SENSING, regarding the client's condition)
- To modify something that currently exists (add, subtract, amplify, distort and otherwise influence that which is already present in the *body*)
- To introduce something new to a system (expose the *body* to colors, waves, vibrations, etc., that were not there before)
- To deliver images, questions and INTENTIONS of other COGNITIVE *skills* to the destination/s established by FOCUS

This is not a definitive list of intentions. It is a sampling of possibilities designed to stimulate your learning.
As you discover other options, add them to the list.

TRANSMITTING is about communicating and connecting, sending out a signal in the form of a thought, image, feeling, idea, intention, color, sound, etc. As intangible *waves*, these signals broadcast, transfer, convey, disseminate, and otherwise make connections. **TRANSMITTING** is the active principle that links the signal to its destination. It is a delivery mechanism and actualizing vehicle for the **COGNITIVE** and other *skills*. It is the bridge between INTENTION and FOCUS.

TRANSMISSIONS can influence the *body* biomechanically, mentally and energetically. Delivering signals, a therapist can highlight and/or modify the current *state* of, or introduce something new, to a system. These signals, which bounce back with information regarding the client's status, are perceived through SENSING. This feedback can be used to make modifications by adding, subtracting, amplifying, distorting or introducing something new to the *body* by **TRANSMITTING** colors, *waves* or vibrations.

PRACTITIONER'S ACTIONS - TRANSMITTING
Use your mental power to send a signal toward a goal and/or have the client do the same.

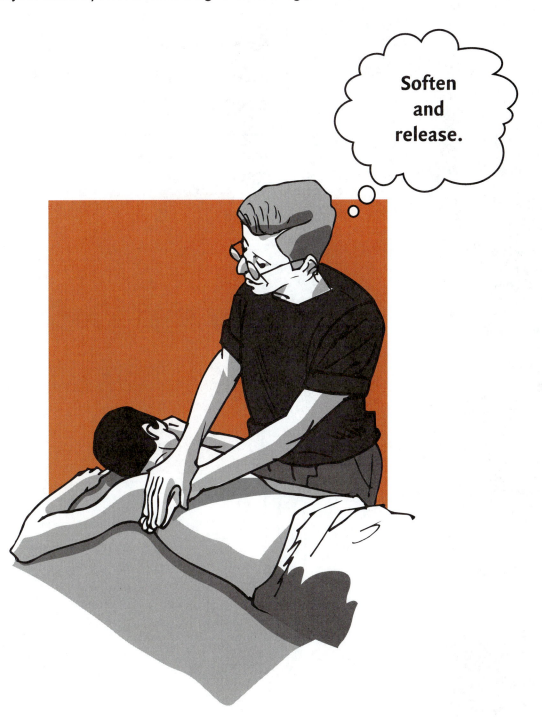

Soften
and
release.

"As surely as we 'call' with our skilled touch, the client 'calls' back and is responding at every moment in a completely unique way.... It is out of the mysterious dialogue of this mostly nonverbal call-and-response that understanding arises. Therefore, the actual practice of therapy has much more to do with the graceful back and forth swing of call-and-response than it does with the unidirectional approach of diagnosis and treatment. When we touch, we are moving within the person's structural body and energy field. Our movements, as we understand the client better and better, become more appropriate responses. When we understand each other, we say we feel in synch."

David Lauterstein,
Massage Therapy Journal,
Fall 1998,
vol.37, no.3, pg.110

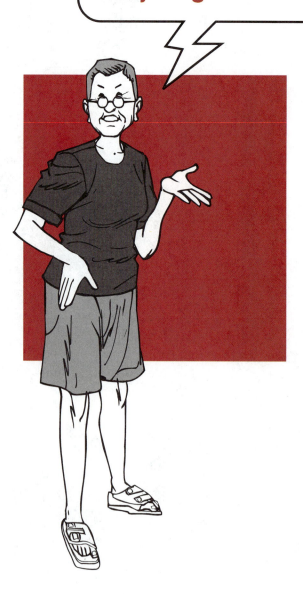

Remember to use this information nonlinearly... everything is connected!

Experientials

Cognitive Component

These exploratory activities are designed to provide a direct experience of the *skills* introduced in this chapter. They are combined and integrated with other *skills* that would naturally occur in an actual *BodyWork* practice. Try them out and observe the results. As you gain proficiency and understand the effects, be inspired to create your own applications.

1. Lift up a leg from behind the knee and in your mind's eye notice how the leg connects to and interfaces with the hip; sense and feel all the way down into the foot.

2. Send a color, thought, feeling or sound to a client.

3. Guide a client to contract and release various muscles throughout his body.

4. Ask a client to create a mental image of what she wants to have happen in a session.

5. Inquire about a client's stress levels regarding work, home, school, relationships.

6. As you mobilize an arm, visualize the joints opening, muscles lengthening, synovial fluid pumping, circulation increasing, temperature changing.

7. With relaxation as the goal, design a plan to treat the head, neck and face.

8. Gently rock a client and focus your attention on her heart chakra.

9. Instruct a client to breathe and visualize a freely moving diaphragm.

10. Formulate an affirmation that empowers the effectiveness of your work.

Modalities Using Cognitive Component Skills

Cognitive Component *skills* can be incorporated into any therapeutic relationship and combined with any *modality*. However, there are *modalities* that feature these *skills* as an integral part of their system.

Some examples are:
Affirmations
Bhakti Energy Work™*
Core Somatic BodyWork*
Cranial Sacral*
Feldenkrais Method™*
Focusing
Hypnosis
Imagery
Lomi Lomi*
Meditation
MDMA®*
PetMassage™*
Progressive Relaxation
Reiki*
Reflexology*
Somatosynthesis
Trager® Approach*
Visualization
Yamuna® Body Logic*
Yamuna® Body Rolling*

*See Linking TouchAbilities®
to Modalities, chapter 23.

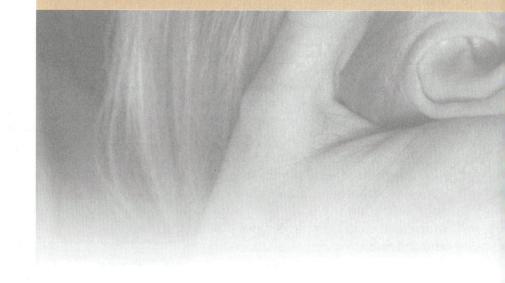

chapter **9**

Energetic Component

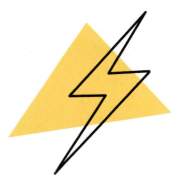

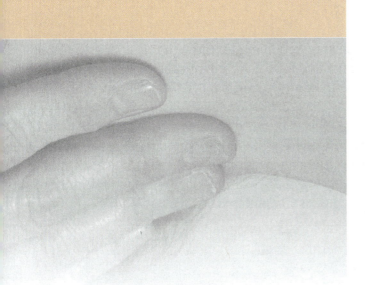

"On the basis of what is now known about the roles of electrical, magnetic, thermal, acoustic, elastic, gravitational and photonic energies in living systems, it appears that there is no single 'life force' or 'healing energy.' Instead, there are many energetic systems in the living body and many ways of influencing them. What we refer to as the 'living state' and as 'health' are all of these systems, both known and unknown, functioning collectively, cooperatively and synergistically. The debate about whether there is such a thing as a 'Healing Energy' or life force is being replaced with the study of the interactions between the biological energy fields, structures and functions."

Jim Oschman, PhD,
Journal of Bodywork and
Movement Therapies,
January 1998, 2 (1), pg. 47

Energetic Component

Introduction

ENERGY is the *carrier wave* of life force. It rides the breath *wave* into and throughout the *body*. Energy animates the *body* and is identified by various cultures as Chi, Ki, Prana, Mana, Orgone, Ruach, Baraka, Kundalini, etc. In his writings, scientist Jim Oshman, PhD, identifies six energetic systems: **elastic, electromagnetic, acoustic, thermal, gravitational** and **photonic**. Practitioners influence these systems by integrating and balancing the *body* in the direction of *homeostasis* by applying the *skills* of **SENSING**, **INTUITING** and **BALANCING**.

ENERGY is expressed in matter through the vitality and *motility* of structure and form. Discordant energy patterns appear in the *body* as stress and distortion. **ENERGY** *skills* are effective in manipulating these distortions and assisting the *body* to establish balance. This is because energetic *fields* are influenced by the many distinctive *wave* patterns inherent in the world. A *body* already in balance can be supported to a higher level of wellness by using these *skills* to expand, maintain and fine-tune currently existing patterns.

SENSING— perceiving or receiving impressions from internal and external stimuli

INTUITING— innately "knowing" through core knowledge or insight: sensing that which is not apparent or visible

BALANCING— supporting, aligning and harmonizing energetic free flow

Sensing: perceiving or receiving impressions from internal and external stimuli

SYNONYMS: perceiving, receiving, touching, tasting, smelling, hearing, feeling, detecting, discerning, being conscious of, being aware of, experiencing

INTENTIONS
- **Electromagnetic system**— To **SENSE** rhythms in the form of pulses (respiratory, circulatory, cranial rhythmic impulse) and waves (brain, breath)
- **Elastic system**— To **SENSE** states of density, tension, distortion, fibrosity, plasticity, resistance, mobility and congestion, and the rhythm of motility.
- **Acoustic system**— To **SENSE** vibrations as expressed through the rhythms of amplitude (range), frequency (timing) and pattern (formation).
- **Thermal system**— To **SENSE** the state of temperature
- **Gravitational system**— To **SENSE** the state of weight, motion, tension and position (alignment)
- **Photonic system**— To **SENSE** color and light

This is not a definitive list of intentions. It is a sampling of possibilities designed to stimulate your learning. As you discover other options, add them to the list.

SENSING is perceiving or receiving impressions from internal or external stimuli. We experience this through our own internal and external **SENSE** mechanisms. Internally, these are our receptors for touch, pressure, pain, temperature and stretch as well as many chemoreceptors that continually function without our conscious awareness. We **SENSE** the external world through the mechanisms of sight, hearing, smell, taste and touch.

It is through proprioception that we **SENSE** the rhythms and states of the electromagnetic, elastic, acoustic, thermal, gravitational and photonic energetic systems. Proprioception is the "awareness of posture, movement and changes in equilibrium and the knowledge of position, weight and resistance of objects in relation to one's own body" (Webster's 3rd New International Dictionary).

Through **SENSING**, a practitioner can feel, detect, discern, experience, i.e., become conscious of the current state of the body. In the electromagnetic system one can **SENSE** rhythms in the form of pulses (respiratory, circulatory, cranial) and waves (brain, breath). In the elastic system one can **SENSE** states of density, tension, distortion, fibrosity, plasticity, resistance, mobility and congestion, and the rhythm of motility. In the acoustic system one can **SENSE** vibrations as expressed through the rhythms of amplitude (range), frequency (timing) and pattern (formation). In the thermal system one can **SENSE** the state of temperature. In the gravitational system one can **SENSE** the state of weight, motion, tension, and position (alignment). And in the photonic system one can **SENSE** color and light (see Chapter 16: SenseAbilities™).

PRACTITIONER'S ACTIONS - SENSING

Use your innate biological mechanisms (sight, touch, smell, hearing, taste, proprioception, etc.) to experience internal and external stimuli.

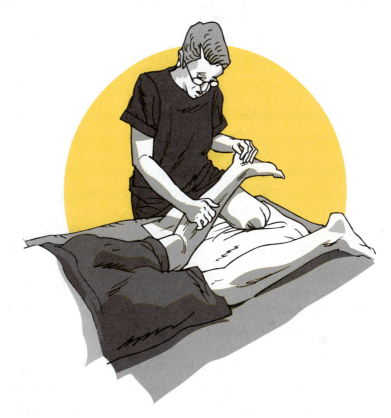

Sensing for shifts in tissue while working the calf

"We naturally take on others' thoughts, feelings, emotions, bodily sensations, images and energy. We live in a shared field of energy.... Just thinking, visualizing or being in the presence of a client, starts an automatic process of exchange between each other.... Clocks, fireflies, menses of women who live in dormitories, the psychophysical moods of husbands and wives, all synchronize their rhythms merely by being in the presence of one another. This is a coupled oscillation. Imagine the coupling that occurs in a healing relationship."

Micheal Shea,
Somatic Psychology for BodyWorkers, 1996

Intuiting: innately "knowing" through core knowledge or insight; sensing that which is not apparent or visible

SYNONYMS: having a direct perception, immediate cognition, hunch, flash of insight, epiphany or inspiration; being in a *state* of "satori"; experiencing a revelation or moment of illumination; having a premonition, impression or gut feeling; operating on instinct; using the sixth sense

INTENTIONS
- To bring subtle knowledge to conscious awareness
- To tap into wisdom beyond logical thought
- To choose applicable *modalities* and *techniques*
- To know when to shift *technique* or place of focus
- To customize speed, *rhythm*, depth, pressure, angle, frequency, location, position, duration, etc., of applications

This is not a definitive list of intentions. It is a sampling of possibilities designed to stimulate your learning. As you discover other options, add them to the list.

INTUITING means "knowing" innately through core knowledge or insight; it is SENSING that which is not apparent or visible. It enables what is known on an unconscious or universal level to be incorporated with and become a part of consciousness. When we know something in this way, we know it suddenly and completely. **INTUITION**, also known as revelation, moment of illumination or premonition, allows for intangible, nonlinear connection and understanding. This kind of direct perception links into truths that extend beyond the predictability of the known. **INTUITION** is often identified as a "gut feeling," an impression, an instinct, a hunch, a "sixth sense," an epiphany, or a flash of insight. This source of inner wisdom leads to clarification and new perspectives.

As practitioners, we use **INTUITION** to "know" which *techniques* to apply, when to shift *techniques* or place of focus, and when to customize speed, alter *rhythm*, change depth, modify pressure, adjust angle, etc.

PRACTITIONER'S ACTIONS - INTUITING
Allow yourself to tap into wisdom emerging from your unconscious.

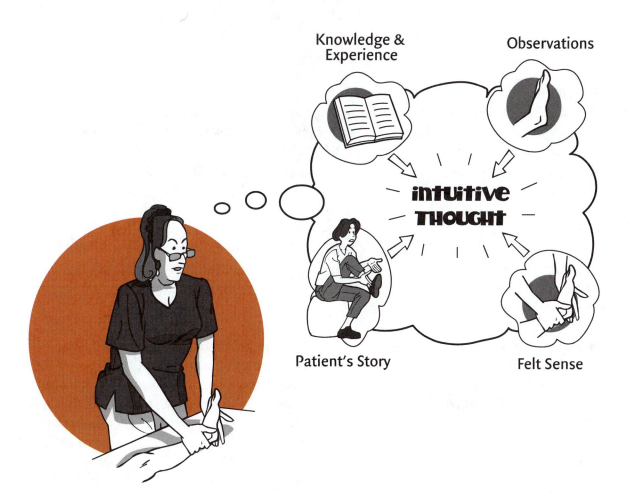

Knowledge & Experience

Observations

intuitive THOUGHT

Patient's Story

Felt Sense

"If you want to be a strongly intuitive being, you don't choose intuition. You choose the elements that build you inside to allow an intuitive voice to come forward."

Carolyn Myss,
Intuition and the Mystical Life, 2003

Balancing: supporting, aligning and harmonizing energetic free flow

SYNONYMS: aligning, harmonizing, connecting, synchronizing, stabilizing, integrating, coordinating, counterpositing, symmetrizing, adjusting, equilibrating, normalizing, correlating, interfacing, interplaying, intercommunicating, interchanging, complementing

INTENTIONS
- To establish *homeostasis* on all levels (physical, emotional, mental and spiritual)
- To support, align, and harmonize energetic flow (within/between chakras, meridians, zones, doshas, elements, paired segments of the *body*, etc.)

This is not a definitive list of intentions. It is a sampling of possibilities designed to stimulate your learning.
As you discover other options, add them to the list.

BALANCE is both a *skill* and a *state*. As a "skill," it is the act of supporting, aligning and harmonizing energetic flow. As a "*state*" it is an energetic experience of support, alignment and harmony. **BALANCING** means to synchronize, stabilize, integrate, connect, coordinate, adjust, equilibrate, normalize, correlate or complement.

Homeostasis refers to the balance of the internal environment of the *body* (microcosm) as well as the *body's* dynamic relationship with the external environment (macrocosm). Using **BALANCE** as an INTENTION, a therapist can assist movement toward *homeostasis* on all levels— physical, emotional, mental and spiritual. The ultimate goal is for optimum function, a smooth interface and a supportive relationship for all *body* parts and processes. Some *modalities* use concepts of chakras, meridians, zones, doshas, elements or paired segments in the *body* as focal points or pathways for **BALANCE**.

PRACTITIONER'S ACTIONS - BALANCING

Use whatever *skills* and capacities you have to influence your client's dynamic nature in the direction of *homeostasis*.

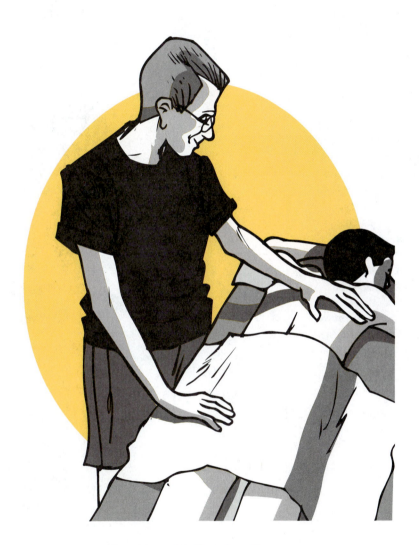

Balancing and influencing client's
energy toward homeostasis

"We live in the world of the third dimension. If one of us lifts up his/her consciousness, they will experience the fourth dimension. The fourth dimension is the world of intuition, the world of higher laws and powers which cannot be measured in a scientific way, because it is of another level. Science is still saying that if something cannot be measured it does not exist. The laws of intuition and spiritual attunement cannot be measured and yet they exist."

Rev. Hanna Kroger,
Help One Another,
2002

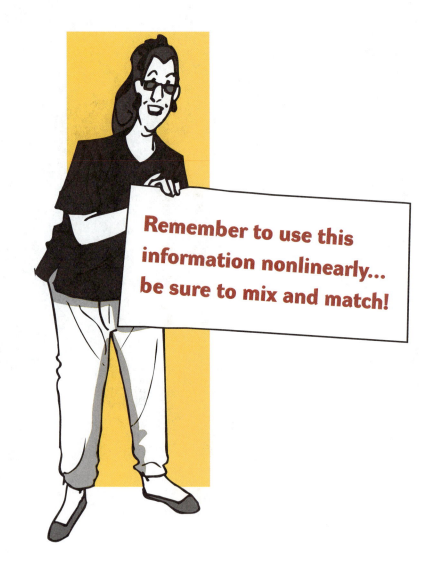

Remember to use this information nonlinearly... be sure to mix and match!

Experientials

Energetic Component

These exploratory activities are designed to provide a direct experience of the *skills* introduced in this chapter. They are combined and integrated with other *skills* that would naturally occur in an actual *BodyWork* practice. Try them out and observe the results. As you gain proficiency and understand the effects, be inspired to create your own applications.

1. Hold a client's head and monitor the infinitesimal movement of the cranial bones.

2. Lift up and feel the weight of an arm; a leg; a shoulder.

3. Explore the surface of a *body* for hot and cold spots.

4. Listen for sounds as you mobilize a joint.

5. Move a client's arm and notice what you pick up about his willingness to be passive and surrender the arm to you.

6. After softly gazing at a *body*, intuitively place your hands where it feels "just right" to work.

7. Lean into the quadriceps and experience how the tissue allows you in or not.

8. Rub a tendon and focus on the changes in length, shape, temperature and size.

9. See what attitudes, history, ideas, traumas or joys you can pick up in a client's energetic field.

10. Place your hands on the crown and heart chakras; sense the energy flow between them and balance it.

Modalities Using Energetic Component Skills

Energy Component *skills* can be incorporated into any therapeutic relationship and combined with any *modality*. However, there are *modalities* that feature these *skills* as an integral part of their system.

Some examples are:
Acupuncture
Acupressure
Amma
Ayurveda
Hydrotherapy*
Inside-Out Paradigm*
Kinergetics
Lomi Lomi*
MDMA®*
Polarity
Reiki
Reflexology
Shiatsu*
Stone Massage*
Thai Massage*
Therapeutic Touch
Watsu
Zero Balancing*

*See Linking TouchAbilities®
to Modalities, chapter 23.

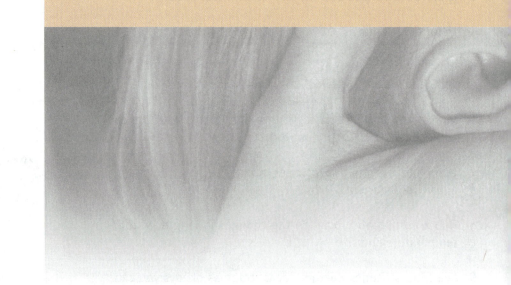

chapter **10**

Compression Component

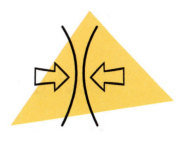

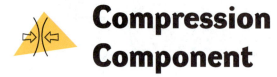

Compression Component

Introduction

COMPRESSION *skills* move energy centripetally toward the core of the target area. The resulting dynamic of interfacing forces and pressures produces *waves* that can be used to stabilize, obstruct, reverse and exaggerate existing *wave* patterns in and beyond the *field of engagement*.

By imposing a force on the *body*, the practitioner influences its inherent flows and moves energy into many directions within and beyond the contact site. These *skills* deal with intentions of distortion, interference, resistance and support. They can be used to explore and assess the *state* of the *body*.

COMPRESSION creates change by challenging defined edges and remodeling shapes and boundaries. Collectively, these *skills* can be used to initiate or assist, as well as obstruct or occlude flows (blood, lymph, energy, etc.). They can initiate, assist and/or resist movement of bones, organs and tissues. They can be used to flatten, stretch, reshape and/or separate *fascia*, muscles, tendons, ligaments and other tissues. Compressive *skills* can also stimulate or override nerve impulses to dissipate trigger points, release contracted muscles and influence neurological patterns.

The degree of pressure varies depending on the density and tension of the tissues being compressed and the intention for the application. It is important to meet and match tissue tension to effectively dissipate force along lines of least resistance.

All the **COMPRESSION** COMPONENT *skills* share a similar set of intentions. The differences in their applications produce variations in outcome. Each *skill*, as presented, is a progressive sophistication of the one preceding it. They all, in some manner, affect the cavities, tubes, tissues, bones, flows and pulses of the *body*. They are identified in this particular way to highlight their subtle differences.

PRESSING/PUSHING

PRESSING—   bearing down, applying pressure to, or putting weight upon

PUSHING—   moving something aside, away or ahead by pressure or contact

SQUEEZING/PINCHING

SQUEEZING—   compressing an object, especially between two forces; closing or tightly pressing together

PINCHING—   focused squeezing between the ends of finger/s and thumb

TWISTING/WRINGING

TWISTING—   using various turning motions on a *body*

WRINGING—   compressing while twisting or squeezing

Pressing/Pushing

PRESSING: bearing down, applying pressure to, or putting weight upon

> **SYNONYMS:** crowding, compressing, crushing, lying on, compacting, condensing, approximating, anchoring

PUSHING: moving something aside, away or ahead by pressure or contact

> **SYNONYMS:** setting in motion, advancing, sweeping, motivating, nudging, propelling, driving, thrusting, shoving, prodding, inserting, intruding

INTENTIONS
- To initiate and/or assist flows
- To obstruct/block flows
- To assess tissue quality (resilience, hardness, fibrosity, *mobility*, tension, resistance, receptivity, strength, etc.)
- To assess energy and energy *field/s*
- To identify tissue layer and depth
- To engage and follow the fluids, tissues, energies, etc.
- To initiate, assist and/or resist movement of bones, organs, tissues, energy, fluids, gases, etc.
- To flatten, stretch, reshape and/or separate *fascia*, muscles, tendons, ligaments and other tissues
- To override nerve impulses
- To release endorphins and enkephalins
- To dissipate energy at tissue lesions (tender points, trigger points, tsubos, cysts, etc.)
- To locate and interact with *fields*, boundaries and torsion patterns

This is not a definitive list of intentions. It is a sampling of possibilities designed to stimulate your learning. As you discover other options, add them to the list.

PRESSING and **PUSHING** are grouped together because of their similarities. They are delineated and presented as two variations because of their differences.

Both of these *skills* involve placing force against material objects or energetic planes. The distinction is found in the delivery of the application. **PRESSING** applies pressure to, puts force upon or bears down onto or into a *body*. It can crowd, compress, crush, lie on, compact, condense, approximate or anchor a target area. **PUSHING**, on the other hand, moves something aside, away or ahead using pressure or contact. It sets in motion, advances, sweeps, motivates, nudges, inserts, prods, intrudes, propels, drives, thrusts or shoves the target area. **PUSHING** is actually horizontal **PRESSING**.

A practitioner might **PRESS** into a fluid vessel, thus occluding it, blocking its flow. **PUSHING** the same structure would move the flow forward, encouraging a draining effect. Energy lines, points or *fields*, as identified by various *modalities*, can be **PRESSED** or **PUSHED** for purposes of sedation, stimulation or balance.

Both *skills* can be used as *assessment* tools to examine tissues and energetic edges for resilience, hardness, fibrosity, *mobility*, tension, resistance, receptivity and strength. They provide *proprioceptive* awareness regarding depth and layers of tissue and energy.

A practitioner can either **PUSH** or **PRESS** to initiate, assist and/or resist movement of bones, organs, tissues, energy, fluids, gases, etc. Depending on the application, these *skills* can stretch, reshape and separate *fascia* with a resultant impact on muscles, ligaments, organs and other structures. **PUSHING** and **PRESSING** can override nerve impulses and dissipate energy at tissue lesions, also known as tender points, trigger points, or tsubos.

"When a bone is compressed or placed under tension, the nonconducting, inorganic crystals that make up 70% of the bone register a minute electrical charge known as the piezoelectric polarity. Compression produces a negative piezoelectrical polarity in the bone, tension a positive one. The bone cells responsible for shaping bones after a fracture use these piezoelectric changes to either lay down or remove bone cells."

Hugh Milne,
The Heart of Listening 2: A Visionary Approach to Craniosacral Work, 1998

PRACTITIONER'S ACTIONS - PRESSING AND PUSHING

PRESSING- Place whatever *body* part/s you're using on the target area of the client's *body*. Stay in one place and lean down into that location using your own *body* weight.

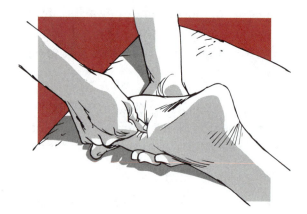

Leaning body weight into the sole of the foot

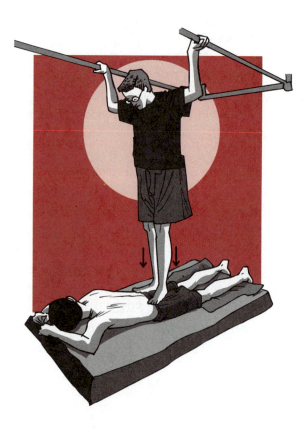

Pressing body weight into the buttocks

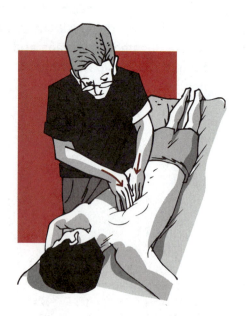

Leaning body weight and effort into the spinal tissues.

PUSHING- Place whatever *body* part/s you're using on the target area of the client's *body*. Lean, using your own *body* weight to produce movement away from the original point of contact.

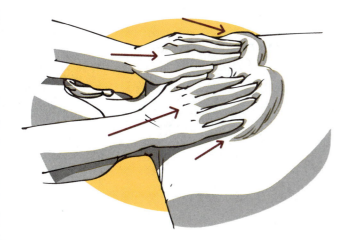

Using body weight to move tissue and energy ahead of hands

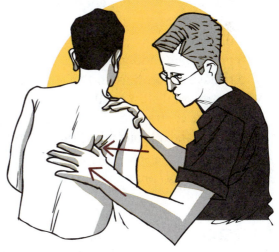

Using body weight to move tissue aside

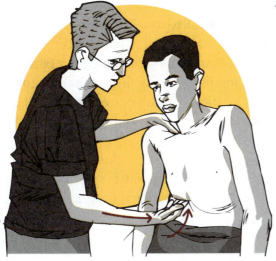

Using body weight to reach up and under the ribs

Squeezing/Pinching

SQUEEZING: compressing, especially between two forces; closing or tightly pressing together

> **SYNONYMS:** compacting, occluding, constricting

PINCHING: focused squeezing between the ends of finger/s and thumb

> **SYNONYMS:** crushing, nipping

INTENTIONS
- To occlude fluid and/or energy flow
- To stimulate nerve response
- To dissipate trigger points
- To pump fluids and gases
- To release endorphins and enkephalins
- To disturb or distort existing fascial and/or energetic patterns
- To release contracted muscles
- To locate and interact with *fields*, boundaries and torsion patterns

This is not a definitive list of intentions. It is a sampling of possibilities designed to stimulate your learning. As you discover other options, add them to the list.

SQUEEZING and **PINCHING** are derivations of PRESSING and PUSHING using opposing forces. They are closely related *skills* with subtle variations in application. In this case, the differences are really a matter of refinement. **SQUEEZING** is the compression of an object between two forces that close or tightly PRESS together. This is accomplished using fingers, palms, entire hand, fists or elbows. This action compacts, occludes or constricts the target area. **PINCHING**, more specifically, is a focused **SQUEEZE** between the ends of finger/s and thumb, as in crushing or nipping.

As with all COMPRESSIVE *skills*, **SQUEEZING** and **PINCHING** affect fluid and gas movement, override nerve impulses, release tissue lesions, assess tissue qualities, affect tissue patterns and impact energy *fields*. Because of a more pointed, specific contact, they are well suited to stimulate the nervous system.

PRACTITIONER'S ACTIONS - SQUEEZING AND PINCHING

SQUEEZING- Place any two of your own *body* parts on opposite sides of the client's target area and move them toward each other.

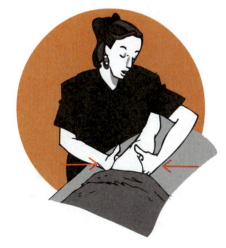

Pressing from both sides to squeeze the thigh

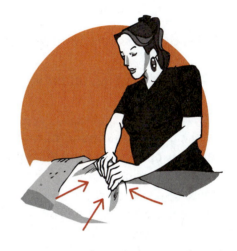

Grasping and squeezing a handful of tissue

PINCHING- Place the tips of your fingers and thumbs on opposite sides of your client's target area and move them toward each other.

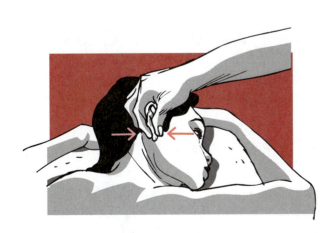

Using fingertips to pinch an earlobe

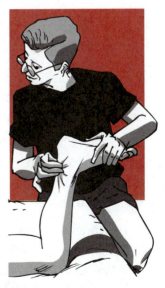

Using fingertips to pinch the Achilles tendon

Twisting/Wringing

TWISTING: **using various turning motions on a body**

> **SYNONYMS:** pivoting, revolving, spiraling, coiling, winding, turning, spinning, rotating, unwinding

WRINGING: **compressing while twisting or squeezing**

> **SYNONYMS:** distorting, contorting, milking, pressing out, expressing

INTENTIONS
- To unlock unconscious patterns and armoring
- To offer new options for functional patterns in tissues
- To create a shearing action
- To create a spiraling action
- To stretch muscle fibers and connective tissues
- To separate fibers
- To challenge and release adhesions
- To distort boundaries
- To stimulate organs

This is not a definitive list of intentions. It is a sampling of possibilities designed to stimulate your learning. As you discover other options, add them to the list.

TWISTING and **WRINGING** add a turning movement to the COMPRESSION COMPONENT. Each one features its own unique style.

TWISTING creates a revolving, winding, rotating *wave* in the *body*. This *wave* can produce shearing forces that stretch, separate and distort layers of tissue, i.e., muscle, organ, *fascia*, etc. It can also involve turning, coiling, pivoting and spinning joints, segments and/or entire *body* parts. It can be used specifically to release unconscious patterns and armoring as well as to challenge and release adhesions.

WRINGING, on the other hand, combines **TWISTING** and SQUEEZING. Specifically, it involves compressing from two opposing sides while **TWISTING**. This combination distorts, contorts, presses out and/or milks a target area.

In addition to the general intentions of COMPRESSION, **TWISTING** and **WRINGING** offer challenges and options to usual, daily movement patterns. Common patterns are primarily along the sagittal plane (flexion and extension). **TWISTING** and **WRINGING** create a shearing action that adds the dimension of rotation in the horizontal plane. They even go beyond that to combine the horizontal plane with the coronal plane to produce spiraling.

PRACTITIONER'S ACTIONS - TWISTING

TWISTING- Use your hands to grasp some point on the client's *body* (either the target area itself or some location in relation to the target area) and apply a turning motion.

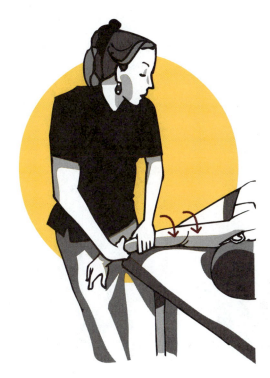

Grasping the forearm to twist the arm at the shoulder

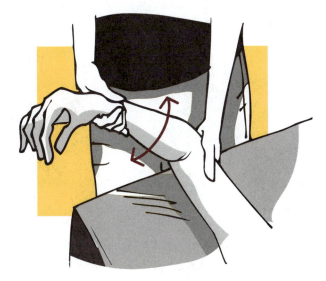

Stabilizing the elbow and twisting the forearm to supinate and pronate

PRACTITIONER'S ACTIONS - WRINGING

WRINGING- Place your hands on two points of a client's target area, compress and move them toward and past each other.

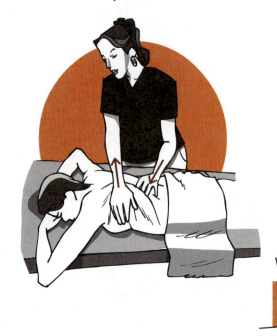

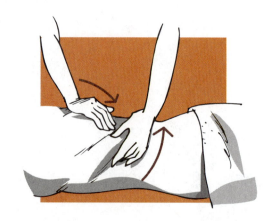

Moving the contact points toward and past each other to create a shearing action across fascia

Experientials

Compression Component

These exploratory activities are designed to provide a direct experience of the *skills* introduced in this chapter. They are combined and integrated with other *skills* that would naturally occur in an actual *BodyWork* practice. Try them out and observe the results. As you gain proficiency and understand the effects, be inspired to create your own applications.

1. Pinch the flesh on a palm.

2. Move lymph by pushing along a lymphatic pathway beginning at the proximal end.

3. Press into a tsubo; muscle belly; origin; insertion; trigger point; energy cyst.

4. Apply a twisting motion to a hip; an ankle; the skin on the forearm.

5. Rotate the head and neck while a client is supine.

6. Compact the space between the metacarpals.

7. Lightly pinch tissue all over the face.

8. Milk the deltoids with squeezing action along its belly.

9. Push the humerus into the glenohumoral joint.

10. Wring the tissues of the inner thigh.

Modalities Using Compression Component Skills

Compression Component *skills* can be incorporated into any therapeutic relationship and combined with any *modality*. However, there are *modalities* that feature these *skills* as an integral part of their system.

Some examples are:
Acupressure
Applied Kinesiology
Amma
Benjamin System of Muscular Therapy*
Chair Massage*
Core Somatic Bodywork*
Cranial Sacral Therapy*
Deep Tissue Sculpting*
Feldenkrais Method™*
Hoshino Therapy®*
Lymphatic Drainage
Medical Massage*
Mother Massage®*
Swedish Massage*
Trigger Point Release
MDMA®*
Muscle Energy Technique
NMT*
Positional Release*
Reflexology*
Shiatsu*
Sports Massage
Structural Integration
Thai Massage*
Yamuna® Body Logic*
Yamuna® Body Rolling*

*See Linking TouchAbilities® to Modalities, chapter 23.

chapter

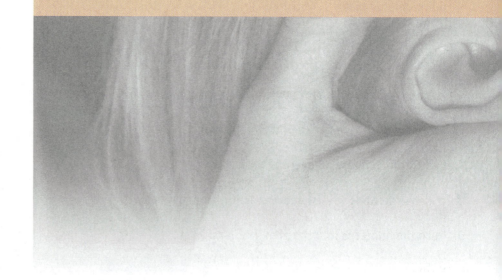

Expansion Component

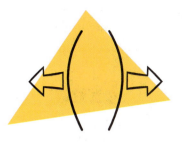

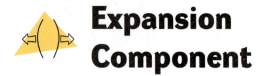

Expansion Component

Introduction

EXPANSION moves in the opposite direction from COMPRESSION. **EXPANSION** *skills* draw matter and energy centrifugally away from the target area. **EXPANSION** and COMPRESSION are complementary and integral to each other. Tissues "expand" around the area of a "compression" and it is typical to grasp tissue with "compression" to accomplish "expansion."

Even though COMPRESSION and **EXPANSION** *skills* are at the opposite ends of a continuum, their intentions and outcomes are similar. These Components are an example of how totally different ways of "handling" the *body* elicit similar results and responses. They can initiate and/or assist flows as well as initiate, assist and/or resist movement of *body* parts. They can also stretch, reshape and/or separate *fascia*, muscles, tendons, ligaments and other tissues. Furthermore, they can stimulate or override nerve impulses, dissipate trigger points, release contracted muscles and influence neurological, energetic and behavioral patterns.

Some distinctions do exist, however. **EXPANSION** *skills* open up the spaces within and between structures. This creates greater *mobility*, relieves impingements and makes room for unobstructed free flow of fluids, gases, energy and information.

The immediate effect of **EXPANSION** is to open and separate structure/s. Its secondary effect is a rebound or trampoline response of tissue or energy bouncing back toward the *body*. The immediate effect of COMPRESSION, on the other hand, is the reduction of space between structures. Its secondary effect is the resultant rebound and "expansion" or opening of these compressed areas.

PULLING—   changing the *state* or condition of, by exerting a tugging force; separating and drawing apart

LIFTING—   raising something from a lower to a higher position; elevating

ROLLING—   lifting and squeezing while mobilizing tissues

Pulling: Changing the state or condition of something by exerting a tugging force; separating and drawing apart

SYNONYMS: tractioning, dragging, drawing, tugging, stretching, lengthening, separating, elongating, opening

INTENTIONS

- To separate tissue layers (skin from muscle, muscle from muscle, muscle from bone, bone from bone)
- To re-establish elasticity in soft tissues
- To stretch and/or separate fibers of muscle and other tissues
- To challenge and release adhesions
- To stimulate organs
- To unlock unconscious patterns and armoring
- To impact energetic *field/s*

This is not a definitive list of intentions. It is a sampling of possibilities designed to stimulate your learning.
As you discover other options, add them to the list.

PULLING creates space by separating, drawing apart, tractioning, opening up and lengthening structures and energies. This is accomplished by exerting a tugging force to change the *state* of the *body*. A possible outcome is to reveal and unlock unconscious patterns and armoring. Structurally, this *skill* addresses the condition and connection of tissue layers. It can be used to stretch, separate and elongate muscle fibers and enhance the elasticity of soft tissues. **PULLING** can separate layers of tissue, i.e., skin from muscle, muscle from muscle, muscle from bone, bone from bone. It can also be used to assess the status of soft tissue and its rebound response, and to expand layers in energetic *field/s*.

PRACTITIONER'S ACTIONS - PULLING

Use your hands to grasp some point on the client's *body* (either the target area itself or some location in relation to the target area) and lean your *body* away from the client's *body*.

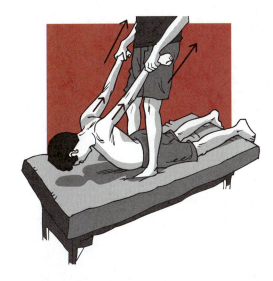

Grabbing the wrists and leaning back to stretch the arms, shoulders, chest and neck

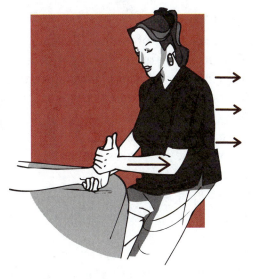

Grasping the foot and leaning back to traction the leg

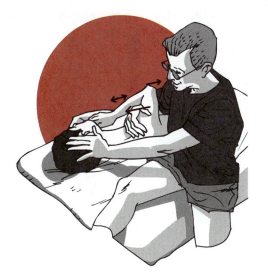

Moving head and shoulder away from each other by simultaneously pulling and pushing in opposite directions

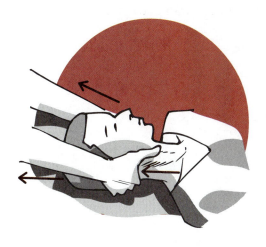

Holding the head and leaning back to elongate the neck

Lifting: raising something from a lower to a higher position; elevating

SYNONYMS: raising, boosting, hoisting, hiking, elevating

INTENTIONS
- To check range of motion (ROM)
- To identify restrictions and patterns of resistance
- To reinforce "allowing" and "surrendering"
- To move or reposition a *body* part
- To feel the weight of a *body* part
- To support circulation
- To promote awareness
- To establish trust

This is not a definitive list of intentions. It is a sampling of possibilities designed to stimulate your learning. As you discover other options, add them to the list.

LIFTING elevates or raises something from a lower to a higher place. Think of boost, hoist and hike. **LIFTING** to reposition a *body* part can create comfort for the client or provide a therapist easier access to a client's *body*. Elevation can also be used to modify circulatory flow, feel the weight of a body part and promote awareness. By **LIFTING** any part of the *body*, a therapist can check range of motion and identify restrictions and patterns of resistance. Through this passive action a practitioner can establish trust and reinforce allowing and surrendering.

PRACTITIONER'S ACTIONS - LIFTING

Place whatever *body* part/s you're using under the target area of the client's *body* and lift. One can also lift a target structure by grasping from above and lifting up.

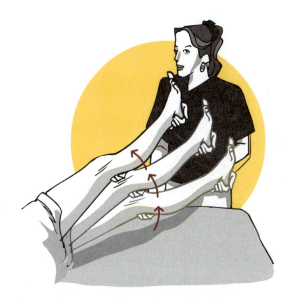

Supporting and raising the leg

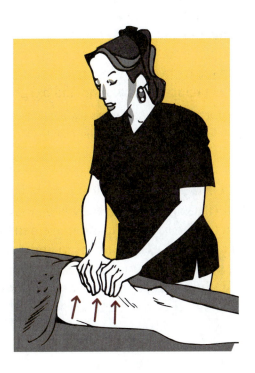

Squeezing a handful of tissue and lifting it away from the bone

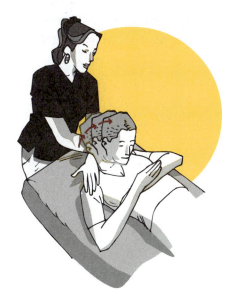

Stabilizing the shoulders while lifting the head with the forearms

Rolling: lifting and squeezing while mobilizing tissues

SYNONYMS: skin rolling, tissue rolling, undulating, turning over, moving in a circular or *wavelike* pattern

INTENTIONS
- To soften *fascia*
- To create greater movement between layers of tissue
- To optimize joint flexibility
- To mold and expand resting options for *fascia*
- To separate, disorient and re-educate layers of tissue
- To create heat
- To encourage circulation and oxygenation of mobilized tissue

This is not a definitive list of intentions. It is a sampling of possibilities designed to stimulate your learning. As you discover other options, add them to the list.

ROLLING is another intricate, *multidimensional skill*. Mechanically, **ROLLING** is a combination of LIFTING and SQUEEZING while mobilizing tissue. It is applied to the skin, tissues and segments of the *body* to expand movement and space between layers of tissue and increase flexibility at joints. **ROLLING** means to undulate, turn over, and move in a circular or *wavelike* pattern. This *skill* is used to mobilize tissue (separate, disorient, and re-educate) and to soften and mold, thereby expanding resting options for *fascia*. Skin and tissue **ROLLING** create heat and encourage circulation and oxygenation of mobilized tissues.

PRACTITIONER'S ACTIONS - ROLLING

Place your hands on the target area of the client's *body*. Squeeze and lift some skin or tissue between your fingers and thumb. Maintaining the lift, roll the tissue by moving your hands in a continuous forward or backward motion. To travel and create momentum, that is, to keep the tissue rolling, your lead digits walk and your following digits scoop under the roll and lift and move in coordination with the lead digits.

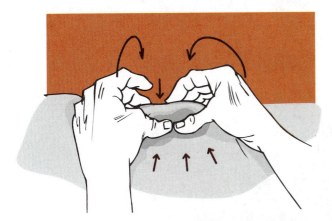

Squeezing tissue and rolling it in a continuous, forward or backward motion

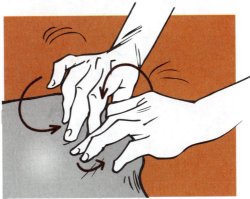

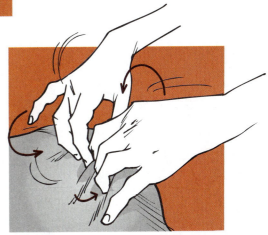

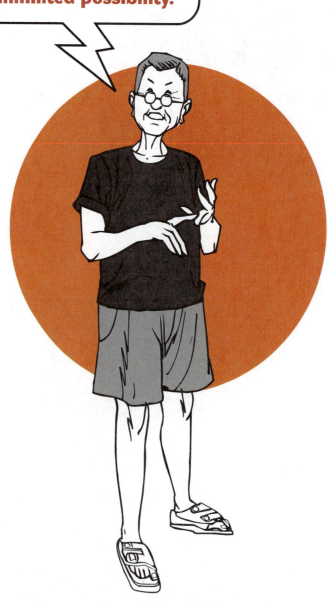

Experientials

Expansion Component

These exploratory activities are designed to provide a direct experience of the *skills* introduced in this chapter. They are combined and integrated with other *skills* that would naturally occur in an actual *BodyWork* practice. Try them out and observe the results. As you gain proficiency and understand the effects, be inspired to create your own applications.

1. Roll the tissue on a back in all directions.

2. Stretch and separate fibers of a biceps muscle.

3. Traction the head away from the shoulders.

4. Roll the skin on the top of a foot.

5. Draw apart the acetabulofemoral joint.

6. Roll the upper trapezius muscle along its anterior edge.

7. Lift and reposition an arm; leg; head.

8. Pull energy out of a knee.

9. Lengthen the quadratus lumborum muscles.

10. Expand a person's auric field.

Modalities Using Expansion Component Skills

Expansion Component *skills* can be incorporated into any therapeutic relationship and combined with any *modality*. However, there are *modalities* that feature these *skills* as an integral part of their system.

Some examples are:
Active Isolated Stretching*
Cranial Sacral Therapy*
Geriatric Massage*
Medical Massage*
MDMA®*
Myofascial Release*
Orthopedic Massage*
Sports Massage
Swedish Massage*
Trager® Approach*
Thai Massage*
Phoenix Rising
Yamuna® Body Logic*
Yamuna® Body Rolling*
Yoga
Zero Balancing*

*See Linking TouchAbilities®
to Modalities, chapter 23.

chapter **12**

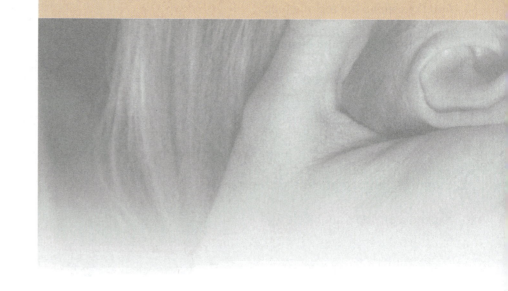

Kinetic Component

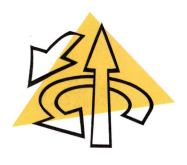

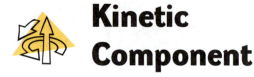

Kinetic Component

Introduction

KINETICS is "a branch of dynamics that deals with the effects of forces upon the motions of material bodies" (Webster's 3rd New International Dictionary). As applied here, **KINETICS** is an umbrella term for a collection of *skills* that focus on the movement relationship between segments of the *body*. INTENTION determines outcomes as these *skills* are used to access information, address conditions and assess treatment progress and effect.

In the subtle realm, this component reveals *body* receptivity to touch and support. Moving on a continuum from stillness to the edge of a client's range of motion, whether active, passive, resistive or assistive, one can assess the *state* of a joint and its surrounding tissues. Is there acceptance of the practitioner's *presence* and holding? Is there fluid *mobility* of the parts consistent with their action potential? Does the articulation feel "dry" or "gritty," perhaps in need of hydration? Are there holding patterns, habitual or otherwise, originating in the physical, mental and/or emotional *fields*? Is the range of motion less than optimal? Are there bony or soft tissue limitations to the movement?

When dysfunction is identified, the therapist may apply the same kinetic *skills* used for *assessment* along with other TouchAbilities® *skills* to provide a therapeutic influence and/or test responsiveness to the work. A therapist might also focus on and explore a healthy structure to modify it by increasing, decreasing or optimizing current capacity and function. Ease and flexibility of movement are the ultimate goals, and can be reached through the *skills* known as **HOLDING/SUPPORTING, MOBILIZING, LETTING GO/DROPPING** and **STABILIZING**.

HOLDING/SUPPORTING

HOLDING— grasping; holding onto

SUPPORTING— bearing the weight of

MOBILIZING— directing and moving *body* parts at joints

LETTING GO/DROPPING

LETTING GO— releasing a hold; loosening a grip on

DROPPING— causing to fall or descend in space

STABILIZING— limiting motion of, maintaining position

Holding/Supporting

HOLDING: grasping; holding onto

SYNONYMS: grasping, gripping, handling, clasping, embracing, cradling, sustaining

SUPPORTING: bearing the weight of

SYNONYMS: bearing, suspending, propping, bolstering, carrying, upholding

INTENTIONS
- To nurture and soothe the spirit
- To release mental, emotional and physical tension
- To stimulate, sedate or reprogram the nervous system
- To take over the effort of muscles in maintaining a *body* position
- To create stillness
- To connect points of energy within the *body*
- To link to higher channels and energy *fields*
- To promote heat transfer
- To access and/or assess the *state* of something

This is not a definitive list of intentions. It is a sampling of possibilities designed to stimulate your learning. As you discover other options, add them to the list.

HOLDING is the act of grasping, cradling or "holding on to." **SUPPORTING** actually bears the weight of, or suspends, a *body* segment. **HOLDING** is gripping, handling, clasping, embracing and sustaining and **SUPPORTING** involves propping, bolstering, carrying or "holding up." These two related *skills* are used to SENSE the structure and the *state* of a person; to connect; to nurture; to assess the client's response to touch.

HOLDING and **SUPPORTING** can create stillness and establish trust. They can also take over the effort of muscles in maintaining a *body* position or posture. A practitioner can "lift" and "take the weight of" a part to identify client habits of allowing and surrendering. This is a vehicle for both therapist and client to experience *proprioceptive* awareness, to educate clients about their *bodies*, bringing consciousness to ingrained patterns.

These *skills* can promote heat transfer and influence the nervous system by stimulating, sedating or reprogramming. They can be used to contact specific points in the *body*, making energetic connections between them and beyond, to integrate with universal energy. Both **HOLDING** and **SUPPORTING** soothe the spirit and encourage the release of mental, emotional and physical tensions.

PRACTITIONER'S ACTIONS - HOLDING AND SUPPORTING

HOLDING- Place whatever *body* part/s you're using onto the target area of the client's *body* and maintain a static contact.

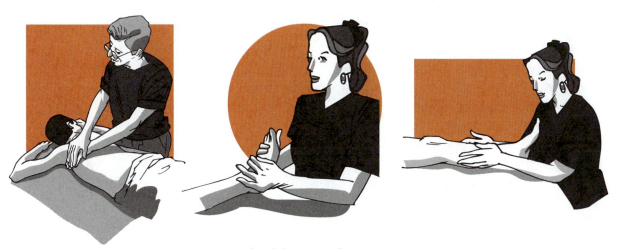

Maintaining a static contact

SUPPORTING- Place whatever *body* part/s you're using under the target area of the client's *body* and exert sufficient effort to bear the weight of the target area.

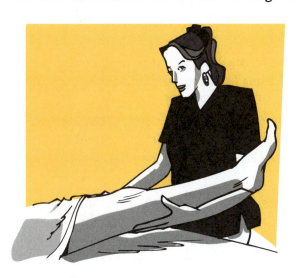

Bearing the weight of the leg

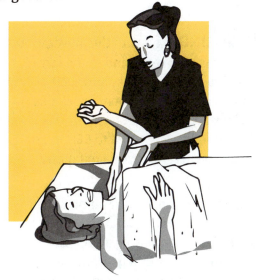

Supporting an arm to establish a specific position

Mobilizing: directing and moving body parts at joints

SYNONYMS: moving, setting in motion, actuating, motivating, activating, raising, lowering, moving side to side, rotating, turning, manipulating, dislodging, exercising, putting into use, shifting position

INTENTIONS
- To qualify, quantify and/or increase ROM
- To assess the *state* of joints and their surrounding tissues
- To remind the *body* of its pattern potential
- To activate proprioceptors
- To assess condition of soft tissues
- To open articulations
- To hydrate joint capsules
- To stretch tissues at joints
- To strengthen muscles
- To tone muscles
- To pump synovial, venous and lymphatic fluids
- To engage and follow fluid, energy and articular motion
- To energize *body* systems

This is not a definitive list of intentions. It is a sampling of possibilities designed to stimulate your learning. As you discover other options, add them to the list.

MOBILIZING plays with the movement potential of the *body*. This ranges from the subtlest, quietest signs of ease or bind to the largest movement currently available at a joint or joints. **MOBILIZING** is a way to assess and treat articulations and their surrounding tissues. This encompasses all manner of movement in any direction, through all planes and elevations, for example, raising, lowering, rotating, pushing, pulling, manipulating, dislodging and moving side to side. This *skill* can be used as a tool to SENSE and identify resistance or restriction in movement patterns. It can also be used to reveal limitations in, and remind the *body* of, its movement potential.

Resisting movement at a joint can be used to assess and build strength and to develop surrounding tissues. Separating bones at articulations lengthens the muscles, tendons and ligaments that surround or attach to those bones. Opening, closing and otherwise manipulating articulations creates a pumping action that stimulates the natural hydration of the joint capsule. This promotes venous, lymphatic and synovial circulation.

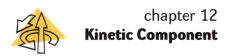
To best utilize **MOBILIZATION**, therapists must have a good working knowledge of the structure and function of the skeletal/articular and muscular systems. They must also have developed the kinesthetic or palpatory sense to recognize, identify and respond to their perceptions. A competent practitioner knows the optimum range of motion (ROM) appropriate for each articular relationship, knows the types of tissues that interface in the joint space and knows the ligamentous structures that bind the skeletal segments together.

The basic **MOBILIZATIONS** are categorized as **active, passive, resistive and assistive**. In **active mobilization** clients move on their own. In **passive mobilization** the therapist moves the client; the client makes no effort. In **resistive mobilization** the therapist offers resistance to the efforts of the client. **Assistive mobilization** involves movement by the client with the help of the therapist.

PRACTITIONER'S ACTIONS - MOBILIZATION

ACTIVE MOBILIZATION- Instruct the client to move his/her own *body* part/s at joint/s.

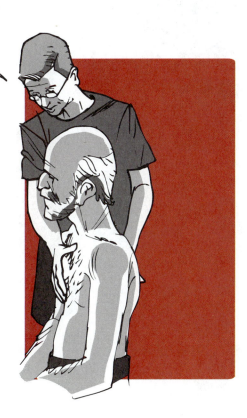

Take in a deep breath to expand and open your rib cage.

PRACTITIONER'S ACTIONS - MOBILIZATION

PASSIVE MOBILIZATION - Take hold of and move the client's *body* part/s at joint/s. (In this instance, the client makes no effort.)

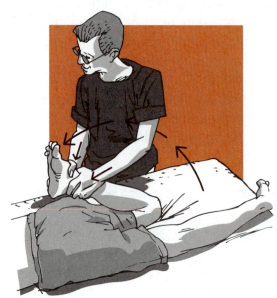

Flexion at the knee

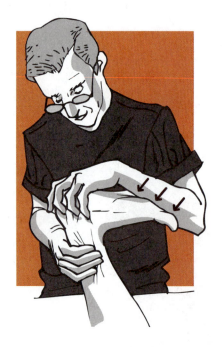

Dorsiflexion at the ankle

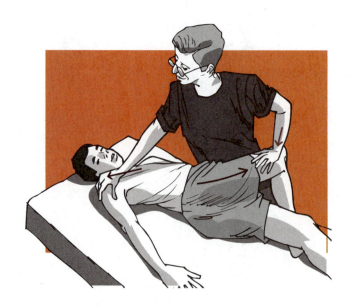

Rotation of the spine

Joint Mobilization Terms

CATEGORIES

Isotonic— muscle tone stays the same; length changes
Isometric— muscle length stays the same; tone changes

TYPES

Active— clients move on their own (isotonic)
Passive— therapist moves the client; the client makes no effort (isotonic)
Resistive— therapist offers resistance to the efforts of the client (isometric or isotonic)
Assistive— involves movement by the client with the help of the therapist (isotonic)

PNF Applications

Proprioceptive Neuromuscular Facilitation (PNF)— This is a collection of techniques that utilize neuromuscular principles to support a therapeutic intention. Listed below are two commonly used PNF techniques. They both employ isometric contraction to achieve a goal.

Post Isometric Relaxation (PIR)
- Target muscle is engaged against resistance.
- Based on the neuromuscular principle that *a muscle will relax to the degree that it contracts*. The target muscle will release after contraction.
  1. Passively stretch target muscle to "soft end feel."
  2. Ask the client to contract target muscle using approximately 10% of his/her strength against your resistance.
  3. Maintain resistance for 10 seconds, then ask client to release contraction.
  4. Use "refractory (relaxation) period" to lengthen target muscle.

Reciprocal Inhibition (RI)
- Reciprocal muscle is engaged against resistance.
- Based on the neuromuscular principle that *when a muscle contracts, the opposite muscle will relax*. As the reciprocal muscle contracts, the target muscle is signaled by the brain to relax.
  1. In most cases, passively stretch target muscle to "soft end feel."
  2. Ask client to contract reciprocal muscle using approximately 10% of his/her strength against your resistance.
  3. Maintain resistance for 10 seconds, then ask client to release contraction.
  4. Use "refractory (relaxation) period" to lengthen target muscle.

"Various kinds of BodyWork and movement therapies can change patterns of movement, and thereby change patterns of electrical fields that arise from that movement, and this ultimately leads to changes in body structure."

Jim Oschman, PhD,
Journal of BodyWork and Movement Therapies,
October 1997,
1(5), pg. 303

"All motion is reciprocal. When you make a motion in one direction, feel what holds you back. What is its size? What is the quality of your holding? What is the quality of your opening?...Where does your body need to bring awareness for balance in the reciprocal tension pattern?

Michael Shea,
Somatic Psychology for BodyWorkers, 1996

Letting Go/Dropping

LETTING GO: releasing a hold; loosening a grip

>**SYNONYMS:** disengaging, surrendering, giving up, yielding, ceasing to hold, relinquishing, releasing, unhanding, unclasping

INTENTIONS
- To complete an intended input
- To move from one place to another
- To allow flow, expansion and rebound from a compression
- To separate energetically
- To disengage or break contact

This is not a definitive list of intentions. It is a sampling of possibilities designed to stimulate your learning. As you discover other options, add them to the list.

LETTING GO is releasing a hold or loosening a grip, that is, disengaging, yielding or unhanding a *body* segment. By **LETTING GO**, a practitioner breaks physical and energetic contact, allowing for repositioning and movement to a different location on the *body*. The act of relinquishing and unclasping might signal the completion of an application. It also permits the flow, expansion and rebound that are secondary effects of a COMPRESSION application.

PRACTITIONER'S ACTIONS - LETTING GO
Release the contact between your *body* part/s and those of your client.

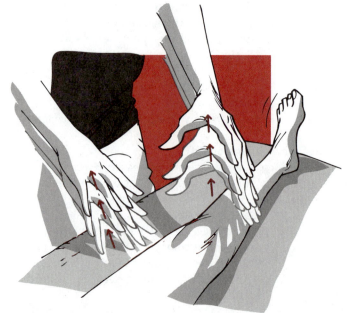

Releasing contact

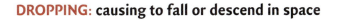
DROPPING: causing to fall or descend in space

SYNONYMS: lowering, letting fall, withdrawing support

INTENTIONS
- To affect *proprioception* through space/time disorientation
- To discover holding patterns in tissues
- To induce and reinforce surrender in/of the *body*
- To free up articulations

This is not a definitive list of intentions. It is a sampling of possibilities designed to stimulate your learning. As you discover other options, add them to the list.

DROPPING allows or causes a structure to fall. It implies that a structure is elevated and the therapist withdraws support, causing it to drop. This is valuable for discovering and challenging holding patterns and/or for inducing "surrender." **DROPPING** can free up articulations and affect *proprioception* through space/time disorientation.

PRACTITIONER'S ACTIONS - DROPPING
From a raised position, remove and release your support of the client's body.

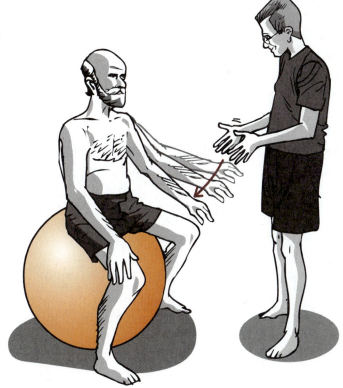

Withdrawing support

Stabilizing: limiting motion of, maintaining position

SYNONYMS: steadying, anchoring, immobilizing, securing, fixing, grounding, maintaining

INTENTIONS
- To create a fulcrum point for motion and leverage
- To limit movement of one part or muscle to allow movement of another part or muscle
- To support *Proprioceptive Neuromuscular Facilitation* (PNF) and other isometric *techniques* (see page 126)
- To facilitate Resistive and Resistive Assistive movements for conditioning, strengthening and rehabilitation (see page 126)

This is not a definitive list of intentions. It is a sampling of possibilities designed to stimulate your learning. As you discover other options, add them to the list.

STABILIZING grounds energy and limits motion. It steadies an articulation. It is used to secure, fix or anchor a joint, creating a fulcrum for motion or leverage. For instance, immobilizing or limiting the movement of one segment or muscle optimizes movement in other areas. **STABILIZING** also allows for the inverse action of a muscle in relation to the typically identified origin and insertion. For example, the upper trapezius muscle typically is identified with elevating the scapula, but if the scapula is stabilized, the trapezius will move the head. Any point or segment of the *body* can be held motionless in order to control and/or direct *mobility* in related tissues.

STABILIZING is core to the use of isometric resistance and specific PNF *techniques* that release tension or increase muscle length. **STABILIZING** can also be used in Resistive and Resistive Assistive MOBILIZATIONS to condition, rehabilitate and strengthen (see page 126).

PRACTITIONER'S ACTIONS - STABILIZING

Place whatever *body* part/s you are using against one side of a target joint on the client's *body* and exert sufficient effort to limit movement.

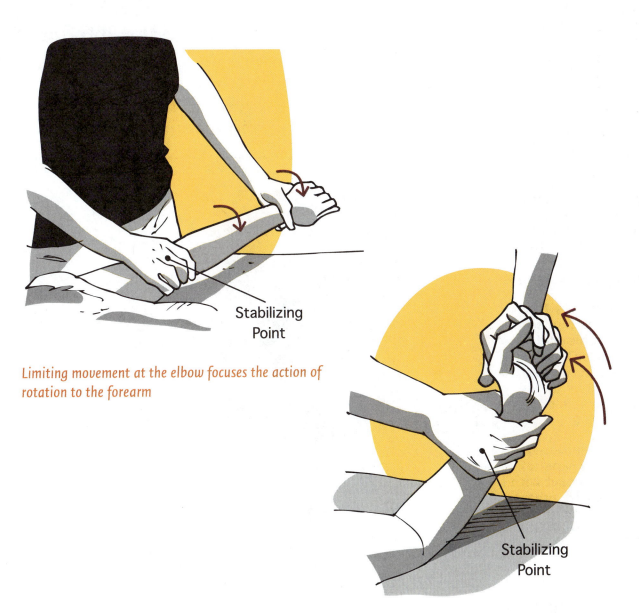

Stabilizing
Point

Limiting movement at the elbow focuses the action of rotation to the forearm

Stabilizing
Point

Limiting movement at the distal end of the forearm focuses hyperextension to the wrist

"Appropriate reactions, the crucial result of clear sensations, accurate perception and the functional organization of accumulated experience, hinge upon three prerequisites within each organism:

1) Free anatomical ranges of motion, unrestricted by habituated limitations or unnecessary defensive inhibitions;

2) The ability to preserve and repeat movements and sequences that have proved in the past to be effective under recognizable conditions; and

3) The additional— and quite separate— ability to react with open-ended, creative flexibility to all sorts of novelties, both enhancing and destructive."

Deane Juhan,
Massage Magazine,
No. 54, pg.56-57

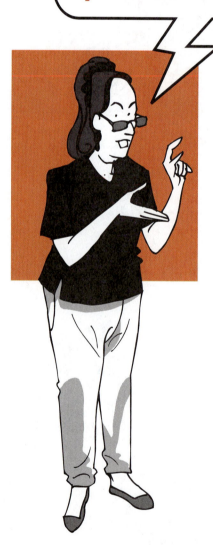

Remember to use this information nonlinearly... the *body* is a dynamic, integrated *multi-dimensional field* of waves, spirals and infinity signs.

Experientials

Kinetic Component

These exploratory activities are designed to provide a direct experience of the *skills* introduced in this chapter. They are combined and integrated with other *skills* that would naturally occur in an actual *BodyWork* practice. Try them out and observe the results. As you gain proficiency and understand the effects, be inspired to create your own applications.

1. Cradle and support a leg; a shoulder; a hip; a hand; a head.

2. Flex/extend/abduct/circumduct an arm.

3. Lift a foot and let it drop down onto the table.

4. Stabilize the top of one shoulder while laterally flexing the head to the opposite side.

5. Provide gentle resistance as a client moves her head from side to side.

6. Make and release contact as you sequentially touch various parts of a back.

7. Use both hands to wrap around and hold a knee.

8. Assist and support movement as a client raises and lowers a body part.

9. Hold a client's arm up in such a way that he lets go of his shoulder joint.

10. Disengage and remove yourself from the field of engagement.

Modalities Using Kinetic Component Skills

Kinetic Component *skills* can be incorporated into any therapeutic relationship and combined with any *modality*. However, there are *modalities* that feature these skills as an integral part of their system.

Some examples are:
Active Isolated Stretching*
Alexander Technique
Benjamin System of BodyWork*
Chi Kung
Connective Tissue Unwinding
Core Somatic BodyWork
Cranial Sacral Therapy*
Feldenkrais Method™*
Hoshino Therapy®*
Inside-Out Paradigm*
Mother Massage®
MDMA®*
Muscle Energy Techniques
Myofascial Release*
NMT*
Orthopedic Massage*
Pilates
PNF
Positional Release*
Sports Massage
Swedish Massage*
Tai Chi
Thai Massage*
Trager® Approach*
Yamuna® Body Logic*
Yamuna® Body Rolling*
Yoga
Zero Balancing

*See Linking TouchAbilities®
to Modalities, chapter 23.

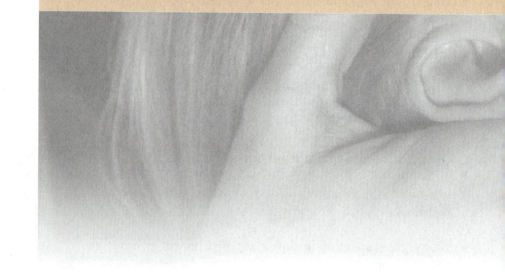

chapter 13

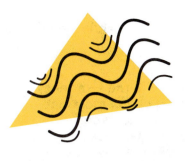

Oscillation
Component

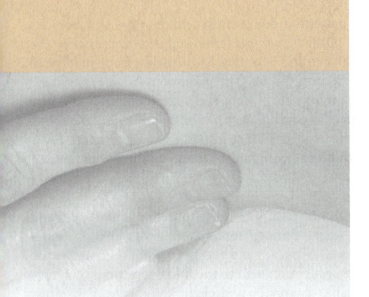

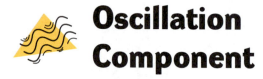

Oscillation Component

Introduction

Everything vibrates and is connected and related to everything else. All matter exists as an expression of, and is distinguished by, its unique oscillation pattern, its vibratory "signature." A healthy *body* is in vibrational harmony. Each aspect of the *body*, material as well as energetic, has its own optimal frequency. **OSCILLATION** *skills* link us with the vibratory *waves* that animate the *body* and all its systems.

Some *wave* patterns produce stress and various disharmonious conditions. Other *wave* patterns support *homeostasis*, the return to balance and harmony. Frequencies, from an internal or external source, can shift the vibrations of an organism— exaggerate, minimize or otherwise alter them. These new *rhythms* affect digestion, respiration, circulation, thoughts, emotions, etc. It is possible to introduce new and/or use existing *waves* to break up rigidity— to loosen, open, soften and align.

OSCILLATIONS initiate reverberation, ripple and rebound responses. As if "surfing," both the client and practitioner "ride the *waves*" of tissues and energetic *fields*. These *waves* run through the *body*, from head to toe, in all directions: horizontally, vertically, diagonally and circumferentially. A therapist extends sensors and feelers to slip into these *waves*, noticing their paths and patterns. Sensations of *rhythm*, flow and swing typify this exploration of motion. What's moving? What's not moving? What feels dull and solid? What feels soft and receptive?

VIBRATING, **SHAKING** and **STRIKING** are the *skills* that make up this component. They are different in form and delivery, yet they each have a similar influence on the *body*—they generate *waves*. Various wavelengths move differently through the *body*.

A small vibratory movement will produce a shorter wavelength and a larger movement creates a longer wavelength. Each part of the *body* is affected differently by the size and frequency of the wavelength.

STRIKING is a staccato *technique* characterized by intermittent and broken contact. In contrast, **VIBRATING** and **SHAKING** maintain continuous contact. Of the two, **VIBRATING** is more subtle, refined and focused, whereas **SHAKING** is a larger, broader movement.

Another distinguishing characteristic of these *skills* is their application trajectory. **SHAKING** and most **VIBRATION** is applied horizontally and the therapist moves along a path parallel to the surface of the *body*. In **STRIKING** the therapist generally moves perpendicular to the surface of the *body*. The action of stationary **VIBRATION** can be both perpendicular and horizontal.

VIBRATING—   applying tremulous, *rhythmic* motion

SHAKING—   moving something side to side; swinging back and forth

STRIKING—   applying intermittent or broken contact, ranging from light to penetrating

Vibrating; Shaking; Striking

VIBRATING: applying tremulous, rhythmic motion

SYNONYMS: pulsating, throbbing, oscillating, trembling

SHAKING: moving something side to side; swinging back and forth

SYNONYMS: jiggling, rocking, swaying, quaking, quivering, fluttering, wobbling, jostling, bouncing, wiggling, waggling, oscillating

STRIKING: applying intermittent or broken contact, ranging from light to penetrating

SYNONYMS: hitting, percussing, banging, cupping, slapping, whacking, smacking, thumping, knocking, rapping, pounding, beating, tapping, hacking, patting, hammering, flicking

INTENTIONS

- To create movement and open joints
- To release holding patterns
- To release emotional holding
- To soften, open and release tissues
- To reduce tension on attachments
- To disorient and reorient *proprioceptive* mechanisms
- To activate, sedate or reprogram the nervous system
- To initiate *rhythms* and *waves*
- To dislodge and release blockages and congestion
- To reveal patterns in tissue
- To nurture and support
- To move stagnant energy
- To penetrate deep into tissues

This is not a definitive list of intentions. It is a sampling of possibilities designed to stimulate your learning. As you discover other options, add them to the list.

VIBRATING, SHAKING AND STRIKING, by their effect, have shared intentions. Individually and collectively, they create radiating *waves* to support a wide variety of goals. These *waves* become signals and patterns of information for every system and every aspect of the *body*.

They all move energy, which can soften tissues and reduce tension on attachments. They all initiate *rhythms* and *waves*. This activates, sedates or reprograms the nervous system, which then can communicate to the *body* to release physical and emotional holding patterns.

As they spread through the *body*, *waves* affect physiology and anatomy. The therapist can shake organs, vibrate muscle spindles, activate proprioceptors, and beat out *rhythms* for support or change. **VIBRATING, SHAKING** or **STRIKING** can tonify, stimulate or sedate organs; reveal existing patterns; create movement and open joints. Oscillation Component *skills* add another dimension to the conversation regarding "attunement" of the *body*.

VIBRATING is the application of tremulous, *rhythmic* motions to the *body*. The *skill* of oscillating can be modified by the various *qualities of touch* such as speed, *rhythm*, duration and intensity. **VIBRATIONS** pulsate, throb and tremble their way through the *body*. As a balancing influence, they may stimulate, sedate or tonify. This action appeals to the *body's* ability to self-regulate, using any and all *waves* and pulses to establish and maintain *homeostasis*.

PRACTITIONER'S ACTIONS - VIBRATING

VIBRATING- Place whatever *body* part/s you're using on the target area of the client's *body* and apply tremulous, *rhythmic* motion.

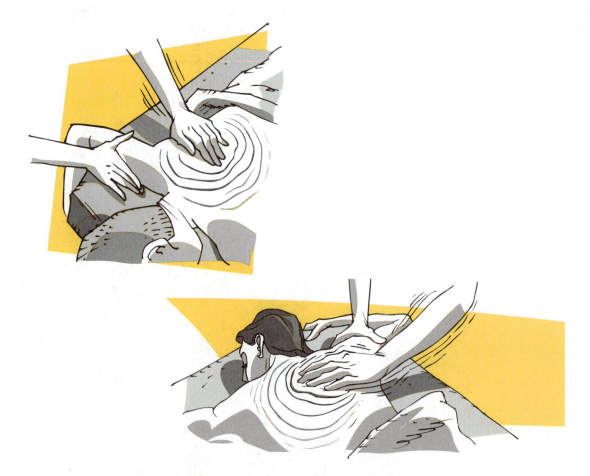

Sending a tremulous motion into the tissues

SHAKING is a gross expression of **VIBRATING**. Imagine jiggle, rock, sway, flutter, jostle, bounce and waggle. These are subtle variations of **SHAKING**. **SHAKING** means moving something side to side and/or swinging it back and forth, with varying speed and intensity. Once again, the overall intention is to engage and harmonize the *body*. With **SHAKING**, one can loosen, soften, open and release holding patterns, congestion, emotions and more. This *skill* introduces *rhythms* that can reveal and reorganize inherent patterns. It can disorient and reorient the *proprioceptive* awareness of tissues and *body* parts. It can move energy along channels and tubes.

PRACTITIONER'S ACTIONS - SHAKING

SHAKING- Place whatever *body* part/s you're using on the target area of the client's *body* and move it *rhythmically* side to side or back and forth.

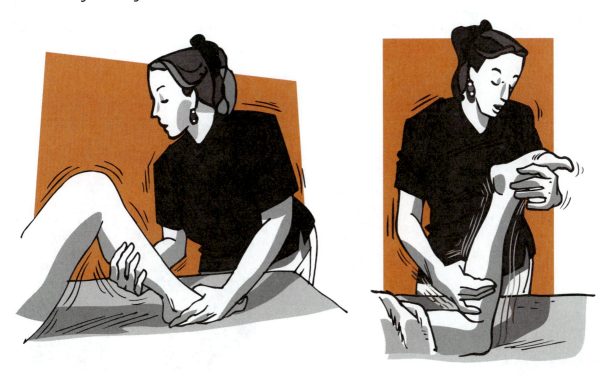

Jostling the calf back and forth

STRIKING is a *skill* that creates *wave* patterns via repetitive broken contact. This intermittent contact, ranging from gentle to strong, sends *waves* radiating from the point of connection. **STRIKING** is like drumming, which creates *rhythms* and *waves* that run like signals throughout the *body*, communicating, entraining, balancing and aligning.

STRIKING is applied with a loose hand. This adds control and *rhythm* to the delivery. The nuances of **STRIKING** are graphically expressed by such actions as hitting, percussing, slapping, thumping, rapping, pounding, beating, tapping, hacking and flicking. **STRIKING** is used, among other things, to stimulate the nervous system, decongest the respiratory system, loosen attachments and create specific *rhythms*.

PRACTITIONER'S ACTIONS - STRIKING

STRIKING- Use part/s of your own *body* (most commonly hands) to make intermittent and broken contact to the target area of your client's *body*.

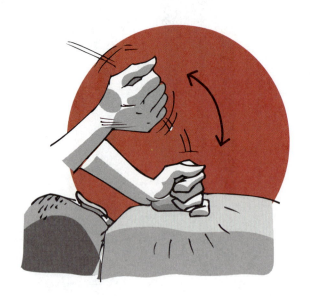 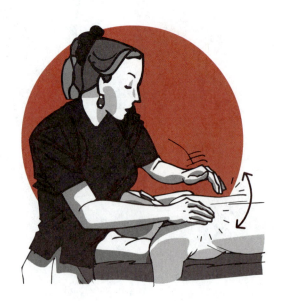

Applying intermittent contact to the back

"We are a series of peristaltic longitudinal and vertical waves.... The first vertical wave involves nutrition and respiration, the internal layer of the tubes. To assist this wave, there are pumping stations – the vaults of the head, the pelvis, the diaphragm of the torso, the hard palate, the tongue, the glottis, the larynx, the pelvic diaphragm as well as the skull and the feet. The next wave connects the nervous system, the internal and external senses, and transports information in and out, up and down.... The next great wave is the support and locomotion of the bones and muscles. Waves of muscle tone support the upright position. The long, slow waves of red muscle fibers close to the spine and the anti-gravitational muscles maintain verticality without effort, while the shorter, more eruptive waves of the white fibers give gestures of immediate response.... The deepest waves are the hormones. They are tied to the blood waves but have a real cyclical outpouring. There are the fast hormonal waves of neurotransmitters and the epinephrine energizers; there are slow waves of thyroid and the pituitary growth hormones....

Pulsatory waves are horizontal as well as vertical, from head to toe. They also have a circumferential flow, like circular rings at right angles to the horizontal flow.... The interaction of the waves, compartments, and diaphragms develops the pressure that resists gravity. All play an important role in uprightness.... Two waves interact – one to push down, one to push up. The feet in conjunction with the ground form a reverberating drum."

Stanley Keleman,
<u>Emotional Anatomy</u>, 1985

"Feeling for rebound becomes clearer through rocking motions. By sensing what bounces back into our hands, we read with great precision where there are gaps or blocks in the flow of movement through the body. We also discover that to accurately perceive the information in the backwash of ripples and waves in another, our own bodies must stay receptive to the flow of waves that we have set up, simultaneously initiating movement and riding it – a skill that requires much practice to master."

Roger Tolle,
Massage Therapy Journal,
Spring 2005,
Vol. 44, No. 1, pg. 67

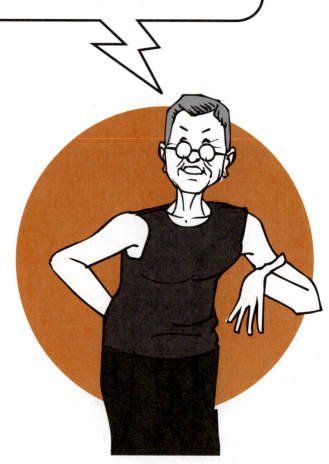

Experientials

Oscillation Component

These exploratory activities are designed to provide a direct experience of the *skills* introduced in this chapter. They are combined and integrated with other *skills* that would naturally occur in an actual *BodyWork* practice. Try them out and observe the results. As you gain proficiency and understand the effects, be inspired to create your own applications.

1. Jiggle a leg; head; shoulder; hand.

2. Shake out a quadriceps muscle.

3. Tap a sternum; iliac crest; maxilla.

4. Beat and soften the fleshy parts of the buttocks.

5. Rhythmically rock an entire *body*.

6. From top to bottom, gently vibrate the spine.

7. Send pulsations through the trunk of the *body*.

8. With a cupped hand, strike an entire back.

9. Vibrate a knee; elbow; ankle; deltoid muscle.

10. Create waves in the auric field.

Modalities Using Oscillation Component Skills

Oscillation Component *skills* can be incorporated into any therapeutic relationship and combined with any *modality*. However, there are *modalities* that feature these *skills* as an integral part of their system.

Some examples are:
Do-In
Dolphin Therapy
Geriatric Massage*
Lomi Lomi*
MDMA®*
Swedish Massage*
Sound Therapy*
Chair Massage*
Trager® Approach*
Water Therapy*
and the use of "tuning forks," light pulsations and electrical frequency machines (vibrators, Vega, Tens)

*See Linking TouchAbilities®
to Modalities, chapter 23.

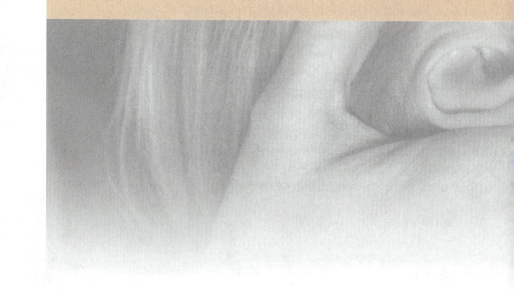

chapter **14**

Gliding Component

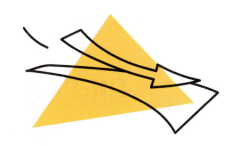

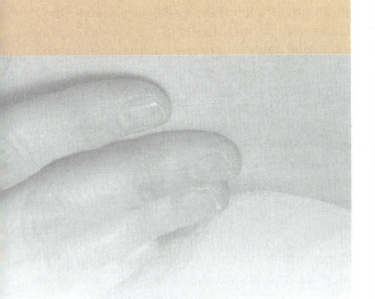

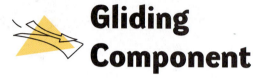

Gliding Component

Introduction

GLIDING *skills* are an interesting mix. The fingers, hands, arms, elbows and feet are used to SENSE and follow the contours of skin, muscle, tendon, ligament and bone. The quality of liquidity in this *skill* allows a practitioner to ride the *waves* of the *body* and experience and transmit a sense of flowing movement. **GLIDING** can be used to sculpt, mold and trace. It can also be used to explore, follow, direct and guide. Whatever the intention, it is truly about the *engagement* of *bodies* in a fluid dance. **GLIDING** is expressed along convergent continuums of opposites: superficial~deep; soft~hard; short~long; fast~slow; *rhythmic*~ erratic; vertical~horizontal~circular, etc.

GLIDING along the skin surface, a practitioner can spread a lubricant, gather information about the general quality of tissues and identify palpable irregularities. **GLIDING** is a tool for locating and distinguishing one type of tissue from another and detecting temperature, texture, tension, density, resistance and shape. It can also be used to affect attitudes and emotions as well as stimulate or sedate the nervous system.

To affect below skin level, a practitioner can engage the *fascia* of descending strata of tissues and **GLIDE** the more superficial layers over the deeper layers. Gradually increasing pressure progressively deepens contact. These *skills* can separate adhesions between and within *body* layers, and release tension patterns to support freedom of movement. **GLIDING** at these levels addresses the subcutaneous *fascia*, intra/intermuscular *fascia*, blood and lymph vessels, tendons, ligaments, all the way down to the periosteum of bone.

In addition to soft tissue influences, **GLIDING** powerfully affects the subtle dimensions of the *body*. It is a specific type of exploration that gives insight into the strength of, and allows *BodyWorkers* to influence vital elements of chi, thermal variation, *wave* pattern and biomagnetic attraction/repulsion.

SLIDING/PLANING

SLIDING— moving across a surface

PLANING— moving along or through subsurface stratum

RUBBING— frictioning over a surface or subsurface stratum

Sliding/Planing; Rubbing

SLIDING: **moving across a surface**

> **SYNONYMS:** soothing, smoothing, slipping, skating, flowing, grazing, glancing, skimming, whisking, brushing, caressing, sweeping, stroking, skidding

PLANING: **moving along or through subsurface stratum**

> **SYNONYMS:** stretching, riding, sliding, flattening, ploughing, ironing, spreading, grading, evening out, leveling, scaling, coasting, carving, sculpting, refining, honing, shaping, burrowing, trenching, following

RUBBING: **frictioning over a surface or subsurface stratum**

> **SYNONYMS:** shining, buffing, frictioning, polishing, spreading, scouring, burnishing, scraping, chafing, scrubbing, scuffing, abrading, grinding

INTENTIONS

- To introduce a therapist's touch to the client (make connection)
- To provide nurturing contact
- To sedate or stimulate nervous system
- To stimulate circulatory and immune systems
- To propel fluids
- To connect parts
- To apply lubricant and other substances to the skin
- To stimulate sebaceous and sudoriferous activity
- To exfoliate skin
- To inspect, palpate and explore the condition of skin or underlying tissues
- To define contours
- To move from one level to another
- To smooth, flatten or level structures and/or energetic *fields*
- To stretch or lengthen tissues
- To create heat
- To separate layers of tissues
- To reduce adhesions
- To soften, expand and open *fascia* and joints
- To promote the release of tension patterns
- To direct, sculpt, shape and/or mold patterns in tissues
- To engage and follow fluid, energy and tissue

This is not a definitive list of intentions. It is a sampling of possibilities designed to stimulate your learning. As you discover other options, add them to the list.

SLIDING and **PLANING** can be used to shape, caress and define *body* parts and contours. They are both powerful tools for *assessment* of texture, temperature, elasticity, skin quality and receptivity to touch. They stimulate, sedate, define, separate, stretch, release, explore, connect, propel and nurture. **SLIDING** and **PLANING** can also be applied off the surface of the material *body* to influence the energetic *field*.

SLIDING delivers the energy of fluidity. The act of **SLIDING** is a continuous glide across a surface. It looks like skating, sculpting, smoothing, soothing, skimming, whisking and swirling. It focuses on moving superficially across the skin. **SLIDING** over bare skin can be enhanced with the use of lubricants. This *skill* is a primary vehicle for nurturing and supportive palliative care.

PRACTITIONER'S ACTIONS - SLIDING

SLIDING- Place whatever *body* part/s you're using on the target area of the client's *body*. Glide on/over the surface of the target area.

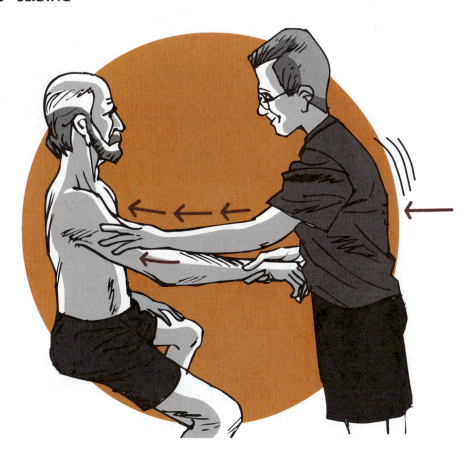

Gliding horizontally across the surface tissue

PLANING moves more deeply into the subcutaneous layers of functional and structural tissue. It looks like stretching, flattening and ironing. It can be used to carve, sculpt, shape, plough, burrow and trench. This deeper action elongates fibers and moves fluids and gases. It advances at varying depths, speeds and angles along the edges of bone and soft tissue. It glides into crevices and fleshy spaces following the directions of muscle fibers and fascial planes. Where it meets resistance in fascial planes it encourages the release of adhesions. This movement is often interspersed with pauses where fascial layers are more glued, dried and disorganized.

PRACTITIONER'S ACTIONS - PLANING

PLANING- Place whatever *body* part/s you're using on the target area of the client's *body*. Glide along any of the subcutaneous layers of tissue. Compress with sufficient effort to engage the target strata or to move through descending levels of tissue.

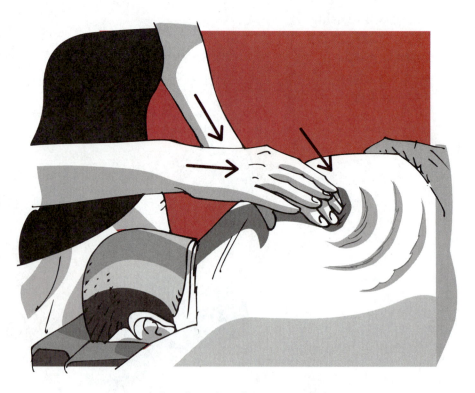

Engaging the subsurface strata of tissue

RUBBING generates heat. Thus it is known within many healing traditions as the "fire-maker." To **RUB** is to move across the surface or subsurface of a structure with friction. This produces different effects depending on depth, angle, direction, speed, *rhythm*, location, etc. Whether gentle or forceful, **RUBBING** ranges from polish and shine to buff, scour and burnish.

Superficial **RUBBING** can be expressed as a chafing or scuffing action as in scratching an itch. It could be a scraping or scrubbing movement to exfoliate the skin or stimulate activity in the sebaceous or sudoriferous glands. On deeper levels, **RUBBING** warms and softens fascial layers and muscle fibers to allow for elongation, separation and greater flexibility. The friction produced by **RUBBING** can soften, reduce or release an adhesion, trigger point or tsubo. It can also affect shifts in tension of emotional, mental and spiritual holding patterns.

PRACTITIONER'S ACTIONS - RUBBING

RUBBING- Place whatever *body* part/s you're using on the target area of the client's *body*. Move back and forth, diagonally or circularly over that surface area, creating friction. For subsurface or deeper layers of tissue, marry your *body* part/s to the surface tissue and slide this layer back and forth, diagonally or circularly over underlying tissue.

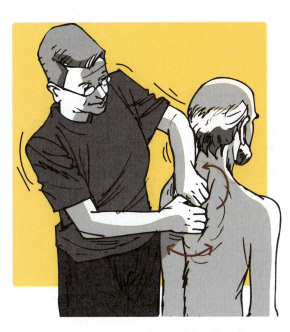

Rubbing across the surface of the rhomboids

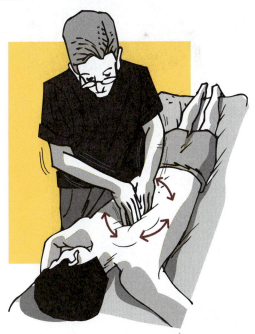

Rubbing deeply into the lamina groove

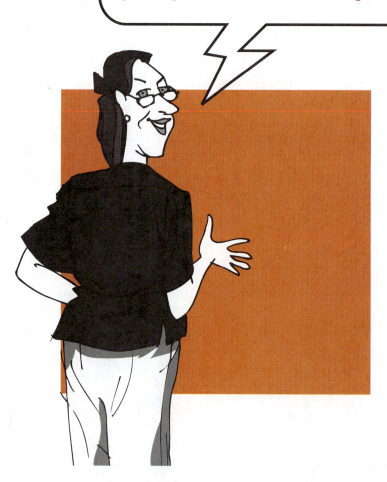

Experientials

Gliding Component

These exploratory activities are designed to provide a direct experience of the *skills* introduced in this chapter. They are combined and integrated with other *skills* that would naturally occur in an actual *BodyWork* practice. Try them out and observe the results. As you gain proficiency and understand the effects, be inspired to create your own applications.

1. Friction around the contours of a joint.

2. Transverse friction the buttocks tissue from superficial to deeper layers.

3. Lightly slide across the superficial tissues of a body.

4. Trace the shape of a foot and toes.

5. Thoroughly rub every inch of a calf; a scapula; the intercostals; a face; a hand; a scalp; an energetic field.

6. Smooth out a nervous system; a chakra; a meridian; an aura.

7. Sculpt the structures of a lower back.

8. Firmly press into and surf the lamina groove of the neck.

9. Plane along the deeper layer of fascia on a forearm.

10. Stroke up and down a spine.

Modalities Using Gliding Component Skills

Gliding Component *skills* can be incorporated into any therapeutic relationship and combined with any *modality*. However, there are *modalities* that feature these *skills* as an integral part of their system.

Some examples are:
Benjamin System of
   Muscular Therapy*
Bhakti Energy Work™*
Chair Massage*
Chua Ka
Cranial Sacral Therapy*
Cyriax Cross-Fiber Friction
Deep Tissue Sculpting*
Hoshino Therapy®*
Lomi Lomi
Lymphatic Massage
MDMA®*
Medical Massage*
Myofascial Release*
NMT*
PetMassage™
Pfrimmer Technique
Rolfing
Shiatsu*
Sports Massage
Stone Massage*
Swedish Massage*
Yamuna® Body Logic*
Yamuna® Body Rolling*

*See Linking TouchAbilities®
to Modalities, chapter 23.

part **III**

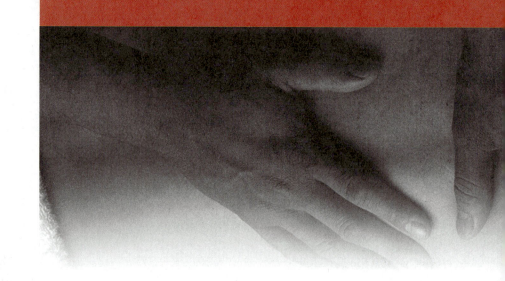

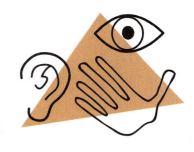

Sensory Experience

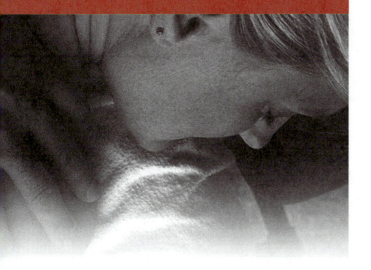

chapter 15

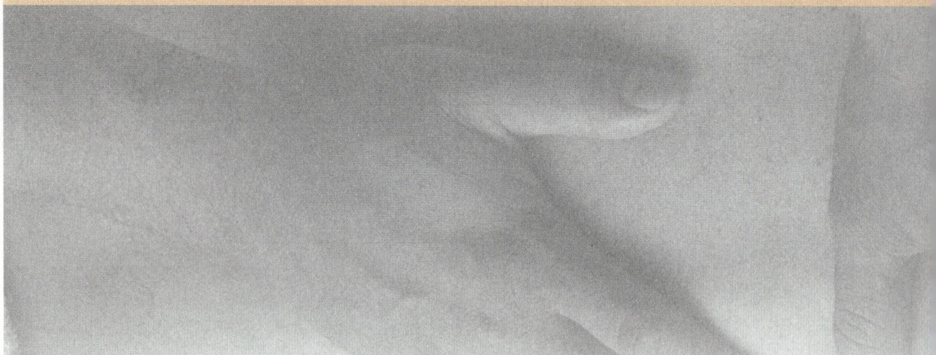

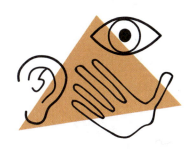

Palpation

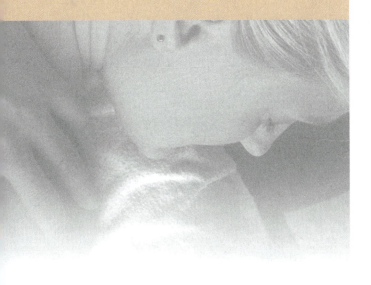

Palpation

touch is contact made from deep within/without
it is that connection transmitted via love and intention
a sense of caring, contribution and relationship
quantum qualities of conscious awareness and personal essence
are the invisible/underlying aspects which drive the action
from an integral perspective creating space, place
the deliciousness of intimacy
center/a state of grace

palpation is to BodyWork as
balance is to riding a bicycle
you do certain things to ride,
i.e., pedal, steer, move thru distance
but there is something beyond the doing
which you must BE in order to actually experience RIDING
it's nothing anyone can give you
it's something you find on your own
thru effort and the desire to ride
it's a state, a way of being that is expressed as balance
balance is finding your horizontal verticality
staying upright against the pull of gravity
it is also a sense of equanimity
center/a state of grace

Exercise for developing palpatory awareness:

- Test the ripeness of a soft fruit
- If the force exerted by exploration exceeds the force within the tissues of the fruit, the flesh will be dented, bruised or ruptured depending on the degree of pressure applied
- Adjusting your force to the forces within the fruit leads to awareness of its texture/maturity/softness and provides knowledge of the state of the fruit

Traditional Perspective

Traditionally, *palpation* is defined as feeling or perceiving through touch. It is the act of pressing on the surface of the *body* to feel underlying structures, organs, tissues, pathways, pulses, etc., in order to identify the size, consistency, texture, tenderness, shape, firmness, location or vitality of something.

Contemporary Perspective

The contemporary version is much more expansive. *BodyWorkers* make contact with more than just their fingers, hands, legs or arms to *palpate*. In the larger view, perception occurs through all of the senses, and goes beyond physical touch. The *multidimensional* client and the *multidimensional* practitioner are completely interfaced and this relationship itself creates a palpable *field of engagement*.

To feel, think and know through the senses is key to being an effective *BodyWorker*. Whether focused on superficial or underlying structures, the fingers (or other *body* parts being used) don't necessarily have to travel very deeply. Rather, practitioners project their sense of touch across distance through varying thicknesses, layers and *fields* of the client's *body* to *proprioceptively* pick up sensations. This information, which comes into the brain through the senses, is just as valid and important as that which is seen directly with the eyes.

As you develop conscious, sensitive, responsive touch, it is important that you approach the body with a "listening hand," that is, use yourself to "stethoscopically" tune into and pick up what the client's body is actually communicating and asking for. Taking the time to "listen" this way will create a session that is in direct relation with, and immediately responsive to, the client. Throughout the session consciously return with a "listening hand" to determine the impact of your work. Be mindful as you gather information, so you can most effectively determine what's called for in the present moment.

"When developing our ability to palpate, there are three aspects to be aware of. First, there is the patient's relationship to, and awareness of, their own body. Second, as practitioners, there is our relationship to, and awareness of our own bodily sensations. And third, there is the interaction between practitioner and patient.... Palpation is a delicate and intimate activity. It involves a subtlety in the nuances of experience in all three of the above aspects. It is a mutual exploration across the boundary between oneself and someone else, an exploration that can lead to discovery and understanding."

Hugh MacPherson,
Journal of Chinese Medicine,
No. 44, Jan 1994, pg. 2

"We will understand better what we feel if we attempt to describe it. In describing what is experienced through palpation we try to classify the characteristics of tissue states, thus not only clarifying our own observations but broadening our collective experience by affording a better means of communication.... We are accustomed to describing crude differences in what we feel by touch, the roughness of a bark of a tree or of a tweed coat, the smoothness of a glass or silk. We must now develop a language of nuances...to apply to palpable tissue states in an effort to describe them accurately."

Paul Van B. Allan, DO, derived from Palpatory Literacy by Leon Chaitow, 1991, pg. 14

Palpation serves as a bridge into the body/mind continuum and between structure and function. It involves perception, discrimination and analysis (aspects of conscious awareness) as well as precision, sensitivity and dexterity (aspects of physical process). This brings to awareness the ways in which the mind is expressed in physicality and how physical states are reflected through the mind.

Proprioception

On the physical level, proprioceptors located in muscle, tendon and fascia throughout the practitioner's body are getting signals and gathering information that makes the experience more than just a local process or even a strictly physical one. When feelings and sensations are picked up and processed through proprioceptive mechanisms, changes of position and tension are registered in the therapist's body. As minute motions are detected, the slightest sensory perceptions are amplified with focused attention. Temperature, density, hydration, tissue layers and so much more can be palpated as practitioners tune into their own bodies to sense the state of the client's body.

Baseline Evaluation

Palpation is a therapeutic tool used for establishing the state of a client's body in a baseline evaluation. It can be a vehicle for teaching people who they are, making them aware of their physical and energetic boundaries, the underlying qualities of their tissue and their bodily sensations such as tension, weight, pain, pleasure, flexibility, surrender and strength.

Monitoring Progress

Palpation is also used to monitor the progress of the therapist's efforts throughout a single session or in multiple sessions over a period of time. Touch is such a powerful healing force, that the palpation itself may simultaneously begin to shift the client's current state. By the time the assessment is over the needed work may be complete.

Guidelines for a more effective palpatory experience:

- Palpate tissue directly, when possible; clothing/draping can interfere with perception

- Relax; tension also blocks perception

- Get clear on the tissue or energy level to be worked

- Approach the *body* with a "listening hand"

- Tune in to the amount of weight necessary to contact the level to be worked on

- Meet the tissue or energy where it is; feel it push back and play with the edges

- Subtly navigate into and out of existing tensions, planes and motions

- Translate findings into meaningful information to guide the work

"Each move is also an invitation – I love this word, it means 'bringing life in' – an invitation to greater awareness, greater movement, greater relaxation. If your hands are suffused with the attitude of invitation as you come into the body, the waves of tension and resistance part in front of you, and depth is more easily found. Entering and waiting, or bringing tissue toward you instead of pushing it, can be a literal expression of this inner 'invitation'."

Tom Myers, Anatomists Corner, Massage & BodyWork, August/September 2004, Vol. xix, No. 4, pg. 90

"...the more muscle tension I have as I work, the less sensitive I am going to be about the changes going on in the client's body. Conversely, the more...relaxed I can be, the more exquisitely I will enter the client's kinesthetic world, feeling the myriad rhythms in the tissues...."

Tom Myers, Anatomists Corner, Massage & BodyWork, August/September 2004, Vol. xix, No. 4, pg. 92

part III
Sensory Experience

Types of Senses
- Touch
- Pressure
- Temperature
- Pain
- Proprioception
- Special Senses- sight, hearing, taste, smell and equilibrium

All sensations involve a receptor organ. Sense receptors convert different types of energy to action potentials, e.g., sound, light, chemical, thermal, mechanical. Receptor responses are specific.

Types of Sensory Receptors and their Functions
- **Exteroceptors**
  - Detect stimuli near the outer surface of the *body*
  - Skin: cold, warmth, touch, pressure
  - Special senses: hearing, vision, taste, smell

- **Interoceptors**
  - Detect stimuli inside the *body*
  - Visceroreceptors: for pH, distension, visceral muscle spasm, pressure, etc.
  - Proprioceptors
    - Found in skeletal muscles, tendons, ligaments, joint capsules; provide a sense of *body* position. For example, Golgi tendon organs are sensitive to tension.

Touch and Pressure
These sense receptors distinguish light contact, deep pressure, vibration and hair movement.
- Light touch: Sensitive to light discriminating touch and low frequency vibration; sensation of something being in contact with the surface of the *body*
  - Receptor organs
    - Meissner's corpuscles detect 20-50 hertz
    - Merkel's disks detect 5-15 hertz
- Firm pressure: Sensitive to high frequency vibration up to 400 hertz; sensation of something pressing on the surface of the *body*
  - Receptor organs
    - Pacinian corpuscles: fast adapting for deep touch
    - Ruffini's corpuscles: slow adapting for deep penetrating touch and skin stretch

Temperature
These sense receptors in the skin detect heat and cold.

> Receptor organs
> - Ruffini's corpuscles detect heat
> - Krause's end bulbs detect cold

Pain
These sense receptors, found in myelinated and unmyelinated nerve fibers, respond to all intense stimuli.

> Receptor organs: nociceptors
> - Myelinated nerves transmit intense, sharp pain
> - Unmyelinated nerves transmit aching and throbbing

Proprioception
These sense receptors, found in skeletal muscles, tendons, ligaments and joint capsules, perceive body position and movement.

> Receptor organs
> - Muscle spindle cells are sensitive to stretch; provide muscle tone
> - Golgi tendon organs are sensitive to tension
> - Joint receptors are sensitive to the position and angle of joints; they provide a sense of *body* position

Smell
The sense organs of olfaction, found in the mucous membranes of the nasal cavity, register odors and smells.

> Receptor organs
> - Olfactory vesicles and cilia are sensitive to air and chemicals

Hearing
The sense organs of hearing, found in the ear, respond to sound waves.

> Receptor organs
> - Tympanic membrane or ear drum responds to sound waves by vibrating
> - Cochlea is receptive to sound waves
> - Organ of Corti: hair cells on this structure convert sound waves to nerve impulses

Equilibrium

The sense organs of equilibrium, found in the ear, respond to movement and weight
  Receptor organs: hair cells located in the following structures:
- Vestibular apparatus responds to position and equilibrium
- Semicircular canals maintain equilibrium

Vision

These sense organs, located in the eyes, respond to light waves.
  Receptors
- Rods and cones, or photoreceptors, convert light to nerve impulses

Taste

Taste buds are the sense organs of gustation. Located on tongue papillae and pharynx, they register salt, sweet, bitter, sour and possibly other basic tastes.
  Receptors
- Gustatory cells or taste buds

"... 'palpation' may also be a harmonic of several senses... detected by the practitioner's hands via mechanoreceptors (Merkel's cells, Meissner's corpuscles, Ruffini's corpuscles, Pacinian corpuscles) and proprioceptors (muscle spindle fibres, Golgi tendon organs). Cutaneous temperature sensors also contribute signals from the site of palpation. Unelucidated sensors may detect brain waves, electrical or magnetic fields, piezoelectricity, or changes in 'body electricity,' as described by yogic practitioners (Green 1983). As Magoun (1976) paraphrased Sutherland, 'This calls for thinking, seeing, feeling, knowing fingers....'"

John M. McPartland, DO, MS, The Journal of BodyWork and Movement Therapies, January 1998, Vol. 2, No. 1, pg. 30

chapter **16**

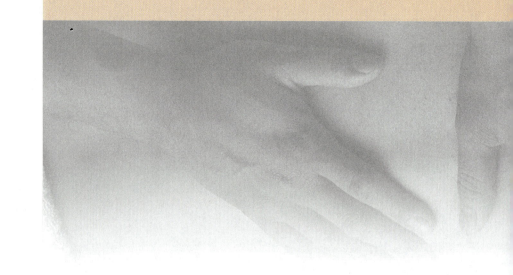

SenseAbilities™

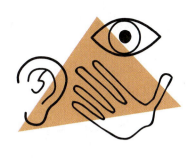

SenseAbilities™

sinking into sensations...

my lean & their resistance...

hardening/softening ~ bending/straightening ~ twisting/winding...

a balance of forces ~ cirque de massage...

the timing/rebounding info feeding into ongoing sensations...

the dance of touch ~ emotion ~ physicality ~ universal mind...

driven thru electromagnetic/piezoelectric messages...

hooking into the rhythms...

every connection is represented by a specific rhythm...

a frequency ~ a cosmic fingerprint flashing into coded sparks of god-light...

it is sensation melding into cosmic continuums...

Introduction

What do you feel when you touch a *body*? How many different ways can you feel? In TouchAbilities® we identify and define *skills* used to interact with the *body*. To optimize the value of these *skills*, it is important to be conscious of what to sense, feel and look for in the *field of engagement*.

By sense, feel and look we mean having awareness of the distinguishing and special qualities of the *body*. The variety of possible sense experiences is what we call *SenseAbilities™*. It represents another link in the interconnected unity of forces at play in a therapeutic session. This realm of interaction enables the therapist to sense and interpret *body* cues, create an intention and respond appropriately.

SenseAbilities™, as a sense vocabulary, identifies and describes experience that promotes awareness for both therapist and client. Each term, word or phrase can conjure up images that become references for communication. Because it is beneficial to clearly describe what is observed and experienced, these descriptive terms can become a valuable point of reference whether writing *S.O.A.P. notes*, session notes or communicating with clients or other professionals.

The following categories are contexts for sensations that might be experienced when engaged in *BodyWork*. Each of these categorical perspectives is presented with possible sensations that define the quality of tissues, energies or emotions that are being focused on during a session.

The *SenseAbilities™* definitions and word listings are part of a dynamic, emerging touch vocabulary. This vocabulary reflects and supports our view on the multidimensionality of *BodyWork* and the *body*. This section is designed to enhance and broaden your touch experience. We encourage you to add other descriptive words not listed here.

Tactile Sense Experiences

Tactile refers to the sense of touch. There are eleven subcategories in this section.

DENSITY refers to the concentration or mass of a substance within an area.

Related Descriptive Words: airy, bloated, bunched, bundled, close, clotted, clumped, clustered, coagulated, compact, compressed, concentrated, concrete, consolidated, congested, choked, clamped, crammed, cramped, crowded, cushioned, decentralized, decompressed, diffused, dispersed, diluted, dissipated, dissolved, empty, firm, full, gathered, hard, heterogeneous, hollow, homogenous, impacted, impenetrable, indurated, jam packed, lumped, scattered, separated, solid, spacious, spread out, stacked, thick, thin.

DEPTH refers to the proprioceptive identification of *body* layers, that is, the awareness of the location of each layer individually and in relation to all other layers.

Related Descriptive Words: bone deep, to the bone, bottom, center, centermost, core, central, cutaneal, deep, dermal, end-feel, exposed, external, fascial, innermost, intermediate, internal, inside, midmost, middle, outermost, outside, overlying, periosteal, shallow, skin deep, surface, subcutaneal, subdermal, superficial, top, underlying, visceral.

FIBROSITY refers to the qualities of tissues that are made up of fibers.

Related Descriptive Words: adhered, attached, braided, bound, connected, crossed, detached, disconnected, filamentous, fibrous, flimsy, fused, gristly, knotted, laced, leathery, limp, ribbony, ropey, scarred, sinewy, strappy, striated, stringy, stuck, tangled, taut, thick, tough, twisted, twined, untwisted, unwound, wiry, wound.

HYDRATION refers to the relative degree of moisture within tissue.

Related Descriptive Words: arid, bloated, boggy, bone dry, clammy, damp, dehydrated, dewy, dissolved, drenched, dried up, drippy, dry, evaporated, flooded, humid, hydrated, liquid, marshy, moist, muggy, oozy, parched, perspired, saturated, seepy, shriveled, sloshy, soaked, soggy, spongy, sticky, swampy, sweaty, swollen, tacky, turgid, viscous, watery, water-logged, weepy, withered, wringing wet.

SHAPE refers to the structural identity of a form.

Related Descriptive Words: angled, arced, arched, bowed, bulbous, branched, bulging, circular, conical, contorted, contoured, crooked, curled, curved, deflated, diamond, disfigured, distended, distorted, elliptical, elongated, fanned, forked, flat, formless, geometric, hairpin, humped, irregular, linear, misshapen, oblong, oval, ovoid, pointed, protruded, recessed, rectangular, regular, rhomboid, round, shapeless, shapely, shriveled, spheroid, spiral, straight, stretched, structured, square, trapezoid, triangular, unstructured, warped.

SIZE refers to magnitude, dimension, volume or bulk.

Related Descriptive Words: ample, asymmetrical, atrophied, big, broad, bulky, contracted, circumference, diameter, dimension, diminutive, dwarfed, enlarged, enormous, exaggerated, expansive, giant, grand, huge, humongous, immense, large, long, magnitude, medium, miniscule, miniature, minute, narrow, obese, peewee, plump, puny, proportioned, rotund, scaled, short, shriveled, shrunken, slight, small, spacious, stunted, thick, thin, tiny, vast, voluminous, wide.

SUPPLENESS refers to the ease and readiness of a form to be bent, twisted, folded, etc.

Related Descriptive Words: adaptable, bendable, bouncy, constricted, contracted, elastic, expansive, firm, flabby, flaccid, flexible, frozen, giving, immoveable, indurated, inflexible, impinged, inelastic, lax, limber, limp, loose, malleable, mobile, moldable, ossified, plastic, pliable, rebounding, resilient, resistant, restricted, rigid, rubbery, sclerotic, soft, splinted, springy, stiff, stretchable, tense, tight, tone, torqued, unyielding, yielding.

TEMPERATURE refers to degrees of hotness or coldness.

Related Descriptive Words: biting, bitter, blazing, boiling, burning, chilly, cold, cool, cutting, fiery, freezing, frigid, frosty, goose-bumped, hot, icy, inflamed, lukewarm, moderate, nippy, penetrating, piercing, radiating, raw, scalding, scorching, searing, shivering, simmering, smoking, smoldering, tepid, warm.

TEXTURE refers to physical and energetic characteristics of the *body*, at any level, from superficial to deep.

Related Descriptive Words: abraded, bumpy, calloused, coarse, coated, cracked, cross-grained, crusted, dimpled, doughy, even, filmy, fine, fluffy, fuzzy, grainy, granular, gravelly, gritty, grooved, hairy, indented, irregular, lined, keloided, knotted, knobby, lumpy, meshed, mottled, mushy, nappy, netlike, nubby, oily, pasty, pimply, pitted, plush, pocked, polished, protruded, ragged, refined, recessed, rough, rocky, satiny, silky, slick, smooth, soft, squashy, squishy, torn, uneven, velvety, webbed, woven, wrinkled.

VITALITY refers to the manifestation or embodiment of vital force on physical, emotional, mental and spiritual levels.

Related Descriptive Words: alert, agitated, attracting, blocked, circulating, compromised, deficient, depressed, ebullient, empty, energized, electric, excessive, excited, fatigued, flowing, frail, full, integrity, magnetism, moving, 'out of synch', pulsating, radiant, radiating, repulsing, robust, scattered, sickly, sinking, sluggish, stable, stagnant, static, strong, surging, vacant, vibrant, vigorous, vital, wiry, weak.

WEIGHT refers to qualities of lightness or heaviness.

Related Descriptive Words: airy, buoyant, dead-weight, ethereal, feather-weight, floating, leaden, light, loaded, hefty, heavy, massive, ponderous, sinking, weightless, weighty.

Visual Sense Experiences

This section includes words relating to bodily expressions, color, complexion and posture. Visual descriptive words for depth, shape, size, texture and vitality are represented within the Tactile Sense Experiences section (pages 170-172).

VISUAL refers to that which can be seen with the eyes. There are four subcategories in this section.

BODY EXPRESSIONS refers to the animation of thoughts and feelings exhibited in the physical *body*.

Related Descriptive Words: attentive, bored, bright-eyed, clenched, contracted, crying, disoriented, excited, focused, frozen, grimacing, glazed over, holding back, impatient, inattentive, jerky, joyous, lethargic, lifeless, nervous, rigid, sleepy, smiling, spasmodic, skittish, staid, stiff, sweaty, tense, teary, trembling, twitchy, unfocused, vacant, wide eyed, wincing.

COLOR refers to the shade or appearance of the skin, eyes, tongue, etc.

Related Descriptive Words: albino, ashen, blanched, black, blonde, blue, blushed, chalky, cyanotic, dark, ebony, erythematic, faded, flushed, gray, indigo, inky, iridescent, jaundiced, light, muddy, olive, opalescent, orange, pale, pearly, pigmented, pink, purple, red, ruddy, scarlet, tan, violet, white, yellow.

COMPLEXION refers to character and quality of the skin.

Related Descriptive Words: acned, anemic, blistered, bloodless, blotchy, burned, bruised, clear, dull, freckled, hyperemic, lackluster, macular, milky, mousy, oozing, pallid, peeling, pimpled, pustular, rashy, rosy, sallow, sanguine, scabby, scaled, shiny, silky, smooth, spotted, stippled, streaky, sunburned, swarthy, variegated, verrucous, washed out.

POSTURE AND FUNCTION refers to the performance and structural relationship of *body* parts.

Related Descriptive Words: abducted, adducted, angled, aligned, anterior, backward, balanced, bent, compensated, crowded, curved, depressed, deviated, distal, distorted, dropped, elevated, erect, even, extended, facilitated, flexed, forward, habitual, hunched over, imbalanced, inferior, injured, misaligned, positioned, posterior, pronated, protracted, proximal, pulled, restricted, retracted, rigid, rooted, rotated, sagging, shuffling, slumped, splinting, superior, supinated, tilted, torqued, twisted, uneven, unsteady, upright.

Auditory Sense Experiences

AUDITORY refers to that which can be heard by the ear.

Related Descriptive Words: arrhythmic, beating, buzzing, choked, clear, clicking, clacking, congested, creaky, crepitating, crepitus, crunchy, distorted, dull, droning, echoing, empty, even, faint, fast, fizzling, flatulent, flowing, fluttering, full, grating, gurgling, growling, halting, hesitating, high, hissing, humming, hollow, loud, low, mellifluous, moaning, muffled, mumbled, open, popping, pounding, pulsing, purring, quiet, rale, raspy, rattling, reedy, rhythmic, rumbling, sharp, sighing, squishy, scraping, scratchy, sniffling, snoring, snorting, squeaky, staccato, strained, strong, surging, thudding, thumping, throbbing, twangy, weak, wheezy, whining, whistling.

Olfactory Sense Experiences

OLFACTORY refers to that which can be smelled by the nose.

Related Descriptive Words: acrid, alcoholic, astringent, ambrosia, aromatic, bitter, briny, decaying, delicate, delicious, fermented, fetid, flowery, foul, fragrant, fruity, gamey, malodorous, moldy, noxious, nutty, nauseating, odorous, piquant, pungent, putrid, rank, rancid, reeking, salty, savory, scented, smelly, smoky, sour, spicy, stale, strong, sugary, sweaty, sweet, tangy, tart.

Psychological Sense Experiences

PSYCHOLOGICAL perception refers to impressions derived from any one or a combination of possible sense experiences. (These reflect *states* of being that are revealed through attitudes and behavior. As we infer, induct and/or intuit, it is prudent to be aware of the potential for *projection, transference* and *counter-transference.*)

Related Descriptive Words: affable, affectionate, afraid, agitated, angry, annoyed, apathetic, appreciative, anxious, armored, bitter, bold, blissful, calm, centered, charged, cheerful, complacent, confident, defensive, detached, distressed, dreary, elated, embarrassed, empowered, energetic, fearful, fragile, gentle, grateful, guarded, grounded, happy, harried, helpless, hopeless, hurt, impatient, indifferent, insecure, integrated, joyful, kind, lethargic, loving, lucid, needy, nervous, open, pained, passive, peaceful, pensive, reactivated, relaxed, satisfied, sad, secure, shy, somber, sorrowful, stressed, submissive, tired, unhappy, upset, worried, wounded

Using SenseAbilities™

The *SenseAbilities*™ foster proprioceptive and intuitive awareness. What do you do with this awareness? What significance does it have for your client? How does it influence your therapeutic response? Consider the following examples of how *SenseAbilities*™ can be incorporated into a *BodyWork* session.

FEEDBACK LOOP

In selecting and applying any *skill* it is essential to maintain a *feedback loop*, that is, to stay open to continuous sensory signals from your client's and your own *body*. In this *state* the interpersonal dynamic supports awareness of any release, shift, change or lack thereof. This, in turn, perpetuates ongoing, constantly interactive connections.

IMAGERY

Sensations can create mental images that may be used as metaphors to trigger and structure ideas for the direction of the treatment. For example, when mobilizing someone's arm, you or your client might get a mental picture of the broken wing of a bird. It really feels like you are holding a broken wing which leads you to treat the person's arm with the delicacy and *skills* required. In this case the visualization serves as a metaphoric tool for healing.

INTUITION

In other instances, sensations can activate or call up impressions and messages that seem to come from nowhere. For example, you can touch a *body* area and get a sense that what you feel there is old. Sometimes you just know when something is emotionally based or when an area is not yet ready to release. This kind of intuitive, intangible information is as valuable as biomechanical knowledge and experience in determining the direction, intentions and *skills* brought to a session.

COMPARISON

Comparison is another method that makes use of sensory information. This occurs on several levels. *Locally*, you compare what you sense in an area with what you know is typical for that area. This means that you need to understand the basic inherent tangible and intangible qualities involved and contrast what you find there with an "ideal scenario." For example, you are working on a client's neck and you know it is considered normal for it to rotate 90 degrees. She can only move hers 45 degrees before she experiences discomfort. So you know that this is an area that needs attention. After working there, the range of motion improves to about 80 degrees, so by comparison you know that you have made progress.

Another way to use comparison is to contrast an area with its *contralateral* counterpart. This provides information regarding polarity and bilateral relationships and influences the direction or focus of the treatment plan. For example, you are working on a client's right shoulder and neck and notice how tight the muscles are. You check the muscles on the left to see if they are tight on both sides or on one side only. This interaction helps to set the direction for the session. You might also look at behavioral influences and ask the client if he carries a heavy briefcase or other object on the right or uses his shoulder to hold the phone to his ear. This conversation just might lead him to change his habits. You can then compare the effects of this change over time.

Yet another perspective involves the wholistic point of view. That is, comparing and interrelating the target area with other *local*, *regional* and *general* areas – from micro to macro. This way of looking sheds light on existing functional relationship and compensation patterns and also influences the overall treatment plan. For example, your client complains of pain in the calf. You observe her walking and discover a pattern that involves the foot, hip and back. Although she may only feel it in the calf, the pattern suggests a broader area of involvement. All of this sets the intention for the work. Comparing the walking pattern during and/or at the end of the session can also be used to measure progress.

Comparison provides an opportunity to look at the relativity of structural and energetic *states* in any number of ways. It's all about organization, relationship and patterns. Consider your findings in regard to such qualities as balance, consistency, distortion, equilibrium, harmony, polarity, proportion, regularity, resonance, symmetry, uniformity, etc.

Whether you are using imagery, intuition, comparison or any other application, effective *BodyWork* is empowered and enhanced by conscious awareness of the messages conveyed through our senses.

"Accessing and practicing tools of feeling rather than doing is at the heart of this work. And I want to teach all of this through their own experience (rather than by talking at them). It is one of the primary principles of Trager to teach new ways of being through repeated felt experience. Massage therapists must have ready access to experiences of lightness, freedom, ease, openness, pleasure and peace in order to share them with their clients. As Milton Trager so often reminded us 'You can only give what you have honestly developed in yourself.'"

Roger Tolle,
Massage Therapy Journal,
Spring 2005,
Vol. 44, No. 1, pg. 62

part **IV**

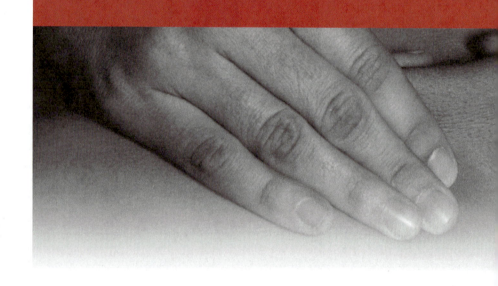

Basic Understandings

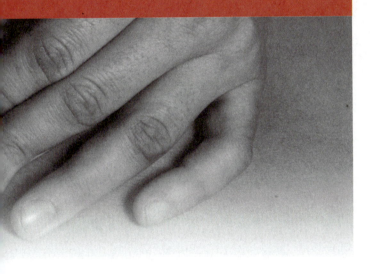

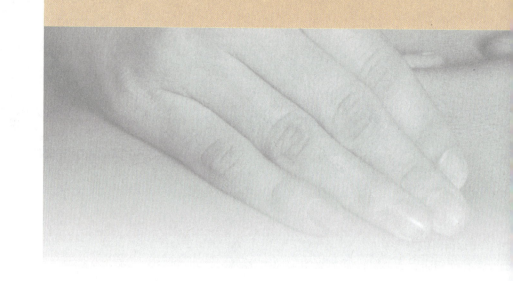

chapter 17

Effects of BodyWork

Effects of BodyWork

Richard Schekter

Introduction

The *body* is an intricate *multidimensional* complex of systems and energy *fields* in constant interaction. It is in a continual process of maintaining balance – internally and externally; micro- and macro-cosmically. This process is known as *homeostasis* and implies that the *body* has an innate intelligence regarding health and optimal function. In other words, the *body* **knows** how to maintain and heal itself. Sometimes, however, external support is needed to restore balance. This might include lifestyle changes regarding personal relationships, exercise, eating habits, medication, stress management and the added stimulus of cleansing, meditation and *BodyWork*.

Challenges to *homeostasis* come in the form of "*stressors*," stimuli or agents that elicit a response from the *body*. Tangible and intangible, these *stressors* can be physical, biological, psychological and socio-cultural. The *body* reacts to these influences with responses that aim to re-establish *homeostasis*. These responses, which we refer to as "effects," occur at all levels— from molecular to *systemic*, from physical to energetic. How the *body* changes in response to these effects is called *adaptation*. Successful *adaptation* leads to a *state* of well-being, increasing resilience and resistance. Poor adaptive responses can lead to *chronic* imbalance, varying degrees of illness and, ultimately, death.

Any change in the external or internal environment, whether positive or negative, may be perceived by the *body* as stress, i.e., an influence requiring a response. In mild doses, the *body* can tolerate, absorb and adapt to these *stressors*. In extended or extreme circumstances any type of stress can be overwhelming and lead to compromised function.

In today's world, stress is typically viewed as a negative influence. Junk food, hostile personal interactions, drugs, air pollution, loneliness, poor health, overwork, excessive exercise and spiteful thoughts, can cause "distress." However, stress can also be seen as positive. Positive stress, known as "*eustress*," might be produced by healthy food, vigorous exercise, friendly interactions, spiritual explorations, and loving thoughts and emotions.

Generally, *BodyWork* as a "*eustressor*" has a positive influence on the *body* and, like other *stressors*, elicits an *adaptive* response. Therapeutic touch exposes the *body* to change and intentionally challenges it to shift toward integration and equilibration.

Factors That Influence a BodyWork Session

Many elements influence the outcome of a *BodyWork* session. We find that paying attention to the following factors makes a big difference in the actual experience and ongoing effects of treatment.

CONNECTION: client/therapist relationship including verbal/nonverbal communication

PRIOR EXPERIENCE: experience and expectation of client and/or practitioner regarding touch and *BodyWork*; *skill* level, knowledge level and *BodyView* approach of the practitioner

PERSONAL PROFILE: biology and biography regarding a client's health history and current health status

ENVIRONMENT: setting (location and equipment), sound, light, temperature, smells and distractions

INTENTION: purpose for session/s created by therapist and/or client; the intention/s may be for the moment, the session or the course of treatment (see chapter 8– Cognitive Component, the *skill* of Intending)

METHODOLOGY: choice of *modalities* and *skills* and the order and frequency in which they are applied; selection of tools and *body* parts used in session; use of lubricant or not; clothed or disrobed client; positioning of client on work surface

QUALITY OF TOUCH: Angle, depth, direction, drag, pressure, *rhythm*, speed and size of application

AREA OF FOCUS: *local*, *regional* and/or *general* parts of the *body* that are the focal point of the application

PRESENCE: focus, awareness and attention of therapist and/or client

DURATION: length of time allotted for treatment/s; length of time spent in one area or with one *technique*

FREQUENCY: impact of one session/cumulative effect of multiple sessions

Perspectives on Effects of BodyWork

BodyWork affects the *multidimensional body* – multidimensionally. Everything is interrelated and interdependent. Touch creates a complex series of interactions and communications that make up what might seem like a singular event. This means the *body* responds simultaneously and sequentially to stimuli on various planes at many levels and stages of development, i.e., physical, emotional, mental and spiritual.

Our "effects" information is primarily based on the written and oral observations and experiences of clients and therapists. Anecdotal lore feeds the knowledge base and provides strong support for what we believe to be the core effects of BodyWork. BodyWorkers and researchers are continually developing methods and gathering data to validate, scientifically and otherwise, the effects of touch. Modern science is now confirming what we have experientially known about the power of *BodyWork*.

Research citations that validate the assertions made in this chapter can be found on pages 329-332. Relating effects to substantiating research is an ongoing process. We invite you to inform us of any other studies that apply to the following statements and/or any effects not included here.

The current understanding regarding the effects of *BodyWork* can be organized and compiled from many different and overlapping perspectives. For our purposes, we have chosen four approaches to the material. The first one categorizes the effects of *BodyWork* in relation to the impact of *techniques* on the *body*. This is represented as *direct* and *indirect* and reflects the nature of the *body*'s responses. The second approach identifies "*general*" *body* responses regarding the impact of touch. The third approach is a systems perspective that is organized in relation to biological organ systems, the manner in which most *BodyWork* students learn about the *body*. The fourth approach features important benefits of *BodyWork* not associated with any particular organ system.

These perspectives are viewpoints from which to see the overall responses that occur in the *body*. They are not absolute and are not particular to any one *modality*. Individual *modalities* identify effects according to their own specific *BodyView* and selection of *techniques*.

The *body* is complex and responds in ways that defy precise inspection and definition. Even with all we know about the function and structure of the *body*, the "how" and "why" of much of it is still a mystery. We are using these categories to support discussion and exploration of the options.

Direct/Indirect Effects

DIRECT—   also referred to as PRIMARY or MECHANICAL

A *direct* effect is the initial consequence of an application of mechanical or energetic forces. It is happening concurrent with and as a result of the interaction between the therapist and the client. This is demonstrated by twisting joints, squeezing tissues, separating fibers, moving fluids, loosening adhesions, etc. It is happening in the moment, concurrent with and as a result of the interaction between the therapist and the client.

INDIRECT—   also referred to as SECONDARY or REFLEX

Indirect effects are the multifaceted physiological and psychological responses to a *direct* application. This application sets into motion a series of reactions, which continue to affect the *body* over time at various levels (physical, emotional, mental, spiritual) and in various locations, sometimes other than that of the initial connection. These reactions are ongoing ripple *effects* of the original application.

Indirect effects are often mediated, i.e., processed, through the nervous system, which stimulates and integrates the natural functions of organs, systems and energy *fields*. Emotional release, reduced tension, stimulation and production of neurotransmitters (serotonin, dopamine), deeper sleep, etc., are examples of *indirect effects*.

General Responses

This perspective focuses on the *body's general* responses to *BodyWork techniques*. These effects can manifest anywhere in the *body* and are commonly part of the *BodyWork* experience. They can occur individually or in conjunction with each other. This is not a comprehensive list; as you discover other responses, add them.

BODYWORK

- Supports *homeostasis* and balance
- Influences fluid, gas and energy flows[1]
- Creates *multidimensional* connections between therapist, client and beyond
- Provides nurturing contact
- Impacts physical, emotional, mental and spiritual patterns
- Improves *motility* and *mobility*
- Releases and/or reduces tension and congestion
- Releases and/or reduces adhesions
- Strengthens and tones tissues
- Restores tissue elasticity
- Produces and/or transfers heat
- Stimulates, sedates, reprograms the nervous system
- Introduces and modifies *rhythms* and *waves*
- Enhances *body* awareness
- Induces relaxation[2, 3, 4]

BodyWork Influences Every System of the Body

To apply *BodyWork* consciously and reliably with therapeutic intent, it is important to understand the *effects* touch *skills* may elicit within or from the *body*. In the upcoming pages we use a system-by-system approach to discuss various *effects*. Although this very linear method provides orderly details and logical sound bites, remember that the *body* is a unified whole and that all parts connect and interact as a functional dynamic. The *body* has an inner intelligence that often responds to touch according to what's needed at that particular time.

MUSCULAR SYSTEM- MUSCLES AND ASSOCIATED CONNECTIVE TISSUE (fascia/tendons)

- Relaxes muscle spasms and relieves tension[5]
- Improves muscle tone[6], strengthens muscles and helps prevent/reduce atrophy
- Stretches and softens muscle fibers, *fascia* and tendons
- Separates muscle fibers and tissue layers to reduce adhesions[7] and fibrosis
- Assists muscle fiber normalization
- Prevents excessive fibrous development and supports unrestricted function
- Reduces accumulation of lactic acid and other metabolites
- Stimulates nerve supply and cell activity of muscles
- Prevents and relieves soreness[8] and stiffness[9] in muscles
- Addresses tender points, trigger points[10] and tight bands and their associated patterns of pain and dysfunction
- Improves elasticity of soft tissue
- Supports ease and efficiency of movement[11]
- Outlines, sculpts and alters contours of tissue
- Improves posture
- Encourages faster healing time for strained muscles and tendons

CARDIOVASCULAR SYSTEM- HEART AND BLOOD VESSELS

- Improves circulation- dilates vessels, relieves congestion in blood vessels and prevents venostasis
- Reduces edema in some cases
- Heightens metabolism and increases *local* tissue perfusion
- Increases transport of nutrients, hormones and metabolic waste throughout the *body*
- Enhances circulation of metabolites into/out of *body* tissue
- Assists venous blood return to the heart
- Constricts and later dilates peripheral arterioles through autonomic effects, creating hyperemia
- Supports temporary reduction or increase of blood pressure[12, 13, 14]
- Reduces heart rate[15, 16]

SKELETAL SYSTEM- BONES AND ARTICULATIONS (including cartilage/ligaments)

- Increases red blood cell production (in bone marrow)
- Encourages retention of minerals (e.g., calcium and phosphorus)
- Assists bone repair
- Encourages synovial fluid production
- Breaks down deposits in joints
- Increases range of motion at joints[17]
- Reduces joint *inflammation* and edema in some cases
- Reduces pain, swelling and formation of scar tissue in sprained ligaments

NERVOUS SYSTEM- BRAIN, SPINAL CORD AND NERVES

- Stimulates *proprioception*:
    - Exteroceptors: through superficial and deep skin pressure, touch and temperature
    - Proprioceptors: affects muscles, tendons, connective tissue tension, stretch kinesthesia
    - Interoceptors: in deeper tissue; affects internal temperature, chemical balance, pH, oxygen and carbon dioxide
- Sedates, stimulates, exhausts nerve impulses/sensations/responses— depending on type or length of treatment
- Reflexively affects internal organs
- Increases endorphin[18] and serotonin production (promotes *states* of well-being and bliss)
- Enhances neurological growth and development
- Encourages hypothalamic balance
- Induces alpha *brainwave* activity, promoting relaxation and creativity
- Induces theta *brainwave* activity, promoting deeper relaxation and problem solving
- Synchronizes *wave* patterns for healing and improved neurological function
- Enhances rest and repair by shifting autonomic nervous system toward parasympathetic activity
- Facilitates and reprograms neurological and neuromuscular patterning
    - Releases and/or reduces physical and emotional holding patterns
    - Releases and/or reduces habitual patterns and armoring
    - Re-educates layers of *fascia* and other tissue
    - Re-educates functional patterns in tissues
    - Reminds the *body* of its pattern potential
- Softens intensity of *body* sensations
- Releases and/or reduces stress
- Relieves and/or reduces tension-related headaches[19, 20] and eye strain
- Reduces anxiety[21, 22, 23]

LYMPHATIC SYSTEM- LYMPH NODES, LYMPH VESSELS AND ASSOCIATED ORGANS
- Stimulates lymph circulation[24, 25, 26]
- Assists elimination of metabolic waste
- Relieves lymphatic congestion
- Reduces edema and lymphedema [27, 28, 29]
- Stimulates immune system[30, 31, 32]

INTEGUMENTARY SYSTEM- SKIN
- Increases blood circulation to the skin
- Raises *local* temperature 2-3 degrees[33]
- Stimulates cleansing and toning
- Activates perspiration and sebaceous gland secretions
- Exfoliates old, dead cells
- Improves texture and appearance
- Increases permeability
- Promotes elasticity
- Reduces scar tissue and scar tissue formation[34, 35, 36]
- Improves nutrition to the skin by application of special lubricants
- Stimulates sensory nerve endings in skin and subcutaneous tissue

URINARY SYSTEM - KIDNEYS AND BLADDER
- Increases urine formation
- Stimulates micturition

RESPIRATORY SYSTEM - LUNGS AND AIR PASSAGES
- Loosens and stimulates movement of mucus
- Increases breathing volume and decreases breathing speed
- Improves respiratory function— can increase air made available to alveoli and decrease work necessary to promote deeper and easier breathing
- Fosters awareness of client's own breath
- Alters breath *wave*, which:
    - Establishes more optimal breathing patterns
    - Connects to the energy of the universe
    - Accesses sacred realms
    - Shifts consciousness and *brainwave* activity (beta, alpha, theta, delta)
    - Influences the *waveform* using diaphragmatic breathing
    - Effects change using the still point between in/out breath
    - Supports self-awareness

DIGESTIVE SYSTEM- FOOD PATHWAY AND ASSOCIATED ORGANS (Mouth, Throat, Esophagus, Stomach, Intestines, Liver, Gallbladder, and Pancreas)
- Increases peristalsis
- Improves absorption of nutrients
- Enhances elimination

ENDOCRINE SYSTEM- GLANDS THAT SECRETE CONTROL SUBSTANCES CALLED HORMONES (Pineal, Hypothalamus, Pituitary, Thyroid, Parathyroid, Thymus, Pancreas, Adrenal, Testes, Ovaries and Placenta)
- Encourages and balances hormonal activity
- Benefits hypothalamic-pituitary-adrenal axis
- Supports positive changes in immune function

REPRODUCTIVE SYSTEM- OVARIES, UTERUS, TESTES AND PROSTATE
- Relieves and/or reduces PMS and menstrual symptoms
- Relieves and/or reduces anxiety associated with menopause
- Enhances circulation to and from the prostate and testes; uterus and ovaries
- Reduces duration of labor[37]
- Reduces morning sickness[38]

Important Benefits of BodyWork not Associated with a Particular Organ System

ENERGETIC INFLUENCES
- Expands energetic *field/s*
- Moves stagnant energy
- Vitalizes life-force energy
- Smoothes energetic *field/s*
- Promotes awareness of energetic systems: (see Energetic Component, Chapter 9)
    - Electromagnetic system
    - Elastic system
    - Acoustic system
    - Thermal system
    - Gravitational system
    - Photonic system

BODY/MIND AWARENESS
- Increases proprioceptive awareness
- Instills a sense of embodiment— self-awareness
- Improves growth and development
- Improves self-image, self-esteem
- Empowers self to make changes
- Brings unconscious material to consciousness
    - Enhances conscious awareness of tension and holding patterns
    - Calls awareness to current *state* of a system/condition
- Defines and redefines boundaries— physical, emotional, mental, spiritual
- Helps access memories
- Helps overcome trauma
- Provides an experience of the *body* as a source of pleasure
- Accesses intuition— taps into wisdom beyond logical thought
- Improves rest and sleep[39]
- Increases attention and concentration (enhances the ability to learn and perform)
- Reduces mental stress and fatigue
- Provides space for "allowing" and "surrendering"
- Promotes a calm/relaxed *state* of alertness
- Fosters trust and provides nurturing, safe touch
- Fosters awareness of mental/emotional *components* of physical sensation
- Expands ideas/understanding
- Enhances ability to monitor and respond to stress signals
- Leads to self-discovery, healing, relaxation, problem solving, insight
- Provides a measure for progress

CONNECTION AND INTEGRATION
- Integrates the "whole" being
- Allows for harmony/resonance between client and therapist; individually within the client; or individually within the therapist
- Connects points on/off/through the *body*
- Links to higher channels and energy *fields*
- Nurtures and soothes the client
- Establishes a communication pathway between client and therapist

chapter **18**

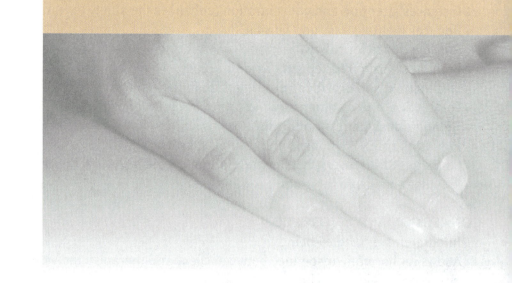

Indications and Contraindications

Indications and Contraindications

Richard Schekter

Introduction

It is essential that a *BodyWork* therapist understand the guiding principles of *Indications* and *Contraindications* to determine if benefit or harm could result from treatment. For the most part, *BodyWork* is supportive of the *body's* process, providing nurturing, balance and improved function. However, applying certain *techniques* to certain conditions could interfere with the healing process, exacerbate the condition or cause the client harm.

Indications

An *indication* is a symptom, condition or particular circumstance that would benefit from a therapeutic procedure. Metaphorically speaking, *indications* are "green lights" to apply *techniques* in response to what a client presents.

Contraindications

A *contraindication* is a symptom, condition or particular circumstance that leads a therapist to cautiously apply or refrain from applying a therapeutic procedure. Metaphorically speaking, this translates to a "yellow light" for caution and a "red light" for avoidance.

When working with a client, ask yourself the following questions:
- Do I have enough information to determine the efficacy of *massage* at this time?
- What questions might I ask the client to become more clear?
- Do I possess the *skills* and knowledge necessary to respond to the client's needs?

If you determine that you are not the right person for the client at this time, ask yourself:
- To whom might I refer him so he gets the care he needs?

This is a challenging subject to address considering the vast *field* of *BodyWork* because it is comprised of so many approaches, e.g., from light energy work to very deep structural work, from gentle easy *techniques* to quite vigorous ones. A particular condition may *indicate* one modality and *contraindicate* another. Sometimes the condition is only *local* (as in the case of sunburned shoulders) and *techniques* may be applied to the rest of the *body*.

Professional Resourcing

In some cases a condition should be treated in coordination with the client's primary health care practitioner. For example, when a client is under the care of a physician, it might be advantageous to check with him or her to determine if the type of *BodyWork* that you plan to perform might have a detrimental impact on the client's condition or the effectiveness of other treatments. Be aware that some physicians are not well informed concerning the effects of *BodyWork*. You may need to learn on your own about the nature of a condition by studying books, searching the Internet, contacting the client's primary health care provider and/or medical specialists, networking with other BodyWorkers, consulting health information agencies, etc., to determine the impact of your work. The physician's lack of knowledge of your particular type of work may necessitate educating them about it before soliciting their judgment regarding the possible effects of its application.

Key Terms

There are some situations that require extra careful attention when considering the most beneficial course of action. If any of the following terms describes a client's condition or situation, it may be necessary to proceed with caution, avoid the area, refrain from treatment at this time, or not provide treatment at all:

Acute— A condition in which the signs and symptoms begin abruptly with marked intensity or sharpness, then subside after a relatively short period of time. Many consider the first 24-48 hours after an injury or onset of a condition to be the *acute* phase. Others refer to the first 72 hours. (This can be an elusive criterion because not all conditions fit within these time frames.) *Acute* can also refer to an intensification phase (i.e., a flare-up or exacerbation) of an ongoing (*chronic*) condition, which then subsides.

Chronic— A condition marked by slow development that persists or recurs over a long period of time; some *chronic* conditions are accompanied by slowly progressing intensification, others by periods of remission and exacerbation.

Contagious— Any condition that may be spread internally through the blood, lymph or other fluid systems, externally along the skin, or interpersonally through breath, touch, *body* fluids or thought. These conditions are often described as transmittable, epidemic, communicable or infectious.

Immunosuppression— Prevention of, or interference with, the *body's* immune responses. It may reflect natural immune unresponsiveness (tolerance), may be artificially induced by chemical, biological or physical agents (e.g., medication for patients receiving organ transplants) or may be caused by disease (e.g., HIV). Decreased immune response increases the *body's* susceptibility to disease.

Autoimmunity— A condition in which the *body's* immune response acts against its own tissues (e.g., Lupus Erythematosus).

Inflammation— Reaction of the tissues to injury, infection or disease. *Inflammation* may be characterized by redness, pain, heat, swelling and/or sometimes loss of function of the injured area. The inflammatory response serves a protective and defensive role. It is nature's way of recycling dead cell fragments as well as neutralizing and destroying toxic agents at the site to prevent their spread to other organs or systems.

Medication conflicts— Medication can cause a *contraindication*, e.g., when painkillers or alcohol affect the ability of a client to give good feedback regarding touch. Blood thinners and anticoagulants make a client more susceptible to hemorrhage. Conversely, *BodyWork* could influence the effects of a medication, e.g., when treatment increases or decreases circulation, it might alter the intended action of a time release pill.

Sensation abnormalities— Heightened sensitivity (hyperesthesia) could limit a person's tolerance for touch or their response to it. Hypoesthesia, diminished sensitivity to stimuli, restricts the client's ability to give accurate feedback on depth, pain or pressure. In either case, failure to modify the *BodyWork* may put the person at risk or cause harm. Certain medications, such as muscle relaxants or painkillers (hypoesthesia), or illnesses such as shingles (hyperesthesia) may cause these *states* of altered sensitivity to touch.

Severe— Describes a condition that is harsh, intense, serious, difficult, extremely strong or powerful.

Systemic— Distinguished from *local*, it refers to something that affects an entire *body* system or the *body* as a whole. This includes any of the physiological, psychological or energetic systems in their individual function or in the way they interface with each other.

Lists and Models

So, is there a definitive list that will clearly identify the *indications* and *contraindications* associated with *BodyWork* for all situations? Of course not! That would be too simplistic. To determine whether *BodyWork* is appropriate, consider the following: the *techniques* to be applied; the symptom/s or condition/s with which a person presents; the physical, mental and spiritual aspects of the client's *body*; and the practitioner's knowledge, *skill* and *scope of practice*. Keep in mind the *body*'s inherent process of continual flux and change. Yesterday, today and tomorrow may call for different things.

Lists of indications and contraindications have been created and appear in some massage textbooks, for example, the Oregon Model and the Ontario Model, featured in <u>Fundamentals of Therapeutic Massage</u> by Sandy Fritz. Such lists can be a good educational starting point, but be sure to identify the approach to the *body* that they represent. Additionally, one man's poison is another man's medicine. For a condition that contraindicates biomechanical applications, energy, bioresonance or *cognitive* therapies might be *indicated*. For example, if a broken bone *contraindicates* working directly upon it, working off the *body* in the etheric *field* or working a contralateral *body* part while visualizing the injured area might be *indicated*.

BodyWork is a valuable *component* of health care, providing elements of nurturing touch and stress reduction, in addition to its many other physical, emotional, mental and spiritual benefits. Most *contraindications* and precautions are based on common sense. Awareness and knowledge of particular conditions are critical for choosing the most appropriate *techniques*. When studying any *modality* it is important to learn the *indications* and *contraindications* relevant to that system.

Some guidelines to consider when applying physical, biomechanical techniques:

- To best support the client's health and cause no harm, it is important to understand the pathogenesis of a condition. For example, if edema is present, know its origin. *BodyWork* might be contraindicated when related to kidney problems, liver disease, venous or lymphatic insufficiency or heart failure.

- When edema indicates *BodyWork*, elevate the affected limb so that gravity assists drainage. Initially avoid working the swollen area and use draining techniques in the nonaffected regions of the body. When intending to relieve congestion as well as improve collateral circulation, it is best to decongest proximal drainage channels before working more distal areas.

- Avoid performing deep *BodyWork* on a client for at least 5 to 7 days following a *severe* injury. Therapy begun too soon could reinstitute bleeding in previously ruptured blood vessels. An exception to this concept would be when there is a physician involved in the case and you are directed to begin work sooner or later than this or advised against working at all.

- With arthritis, do not work on a joint that presents with heat, redness or active swelling (*acute* stage). In the *chronic* stage, when the inflammation subsides and pain is gone, more vigorous kneading and deep friction can be used to reduce the risk of adhesions and restore circulation and muscle integrity.

- Be sure that you understand the anatomy involved as well as a physician's recommendations where there is a loss of integrity in an area, e.g., recent surgery, joint replacement, *severe* rheumatoid arthritis, nonunion fracture, herniated discs, most hernias and dislocations.

Some guidelines to consider when applying energy techniques:

Written with help from Lisa VanOstrand

- It is important to be aware of the psychological and mental *state* of a client. Be cautious about using energy work with people with *severe* mental conditions such as psychosis, schizophrenia or delusional tendencies. This also applies to people who are taking psychotropic medications and drugs. Because these are nonstable *states*, energy *techniques* may trigger and activate unwanted responses.

- Be knowledgeable from a medical perspective about *chronic* conditions or illnesses such as cancer and heart disease. These illnesses may be stimulated or aggravated by energy work.

- Unless you have adequate experience working with pregnancy, avoid doing energy work with the first three chakras during the first trimester. It is possible to stimulate a miscarriage.

- Be alert to a client's mental and emotional readiness to receive *BodyWork* and his/her willingness to deal psychologically with what comes up. If the client is resistant, your work could have negative effects.

- Be sensitive to signs from the *body* regarding receptivity to, and acceptance of, energy work. For some people, this kind of *BodyWork* could be too stimulating or sedating.

- Be realistic about your competency and readiness as a practitioner to handle your own energy and the energy that arises as a result of doing energy work. You do not want to activate, release and/or intensify something you aren't prepared to handle.

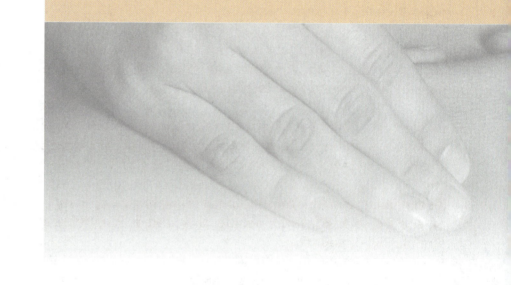

Endangerment Sites

Endangerment Sites

Richard Schekter

In alignment with our ongoing suggestions about working within your *scope of practice*, knowledge, *skill*, etc., be aware that *BodyWork* has the potential to be harmful. The term *"endangerment site"* refers to a *body's* especially vulnerable, delicate or exposed physical locations. These involve delicate tissues and structures such as nerves, blood vessels, and lymph nodes or other organs unprotected by bone, muscle or connective tissue, that could be in danger from pinching, pinning, occluding or entrapment.

"Endangerment" doesn't mean don't go there; it means be aware that these areas are more fragile than others. It is important to know the anatomy and physiology of the focus area: the pathway of vessels and nerves, the lay of muscles, the direction of fibers and the organs that may be present. It is up to you to determine if the work that you do will in any way compromise the structures there. Where there is concern, be more sensitive and either modify your approach or avoid the area.

Some general suggestions when working in an endangerment area:

- Determine the state or condition of an organ or area before proceeding

- Use pressure most appropriate for the condition and design of an area

- Work using angles that most effectively navigate the anatomy of an area

The following chart covers basic *endangerment sites*, identifies the anatomical area involved and the associated endangered structures. There are also notes regarding cautions and considerations when working these areas. For more detailed explanations refer to A Massage Therapist's Guide to Pathology, 3rd Edition, by Ruth Werner.

Endangerment Sites

Area of Concern	Location and Description	Endangered Structures	Comments
Temporal area	- Slightly depressed area over the sphenoid bone	- Temporal artery - Temporal branches of facial nerve - Branches of trigeminal nerve - Trigeminal ganglion	- Excess pressure at the temple may be uncomfortable.
Eye	- Area within the bony orbit	- Eyeball and conjunctiva	- Avoid direct contact with eye or conjunctiva. - Avoid undue intraocular pressure. - Avoid infection or irritation (from lubricants, contact lenses, etc.).
Mouth	- Oral cavity	- Oral mucosa	- Intraoral massage should be performed by trained persons. Imprudent work can cause serious infection, gagging, and harm to both therapist and client.
Temporomandibular joint (TMJ)	- Juncture between mandible and temporal bones including fibrocartilage disc	- Parotid gland - Trigeminal nerve - Trigeminal ganglion - Facial nerve - Superficial temporal artery	- Position of jaw may affect exposure of nerves. - Compressing or damaging nerves may cause trigeminal neuralgia.
Mastoid	- Medial to lower earlobe - Anterior to mastoid process of temporal bone - Posterior to mandibular ramus	- Styloid process of temporal bone - Internal carotid artery - Facial nerve - Superficial temporal artery - Posterior auricular nerve - Posterior auricular artery	- Excessive pressure could damage the styloid process.

Endangerment Sites (continued)

Area of Concern	Location and Description	Endangered Structures	Comments
Occipital area	- Posterior base of skull	- Suboccipital nerve (C1) - Greater occipital nerve (C2) - Third occipital nerve (C3) - Vertebral artery	- Static pressure may be effective. - Digging too deeply could entrap these structures.
Anterior triangle of the neck	Boundaries: - Medial aspect of Sternocleidomasotoid (SCM), bilaterally - Inferior edge of mandible - Superior edge of sternum	- Carotid arteries - Carotid sinuses - Internal jugular veins - Thyroid gland - Hyoid bone - Submandibular salivary glands - Trachea - Lymph nodes	- Pressure on carotid sinus can reflexively lower blood pressure, or diminish blood supply to head, causing dizziness or blackout. - Many lymph nodes are located in this area; especially just anterior to SCM.
Posterolateral triangle of the neck	Boundaries: - Posterior aspect of SCM - Clavicle - Anterior upper part of Trapezius	- External jugular veins - Cervical transverse processes - Brachial plexus - Cervical plexus (in part) - Subclavian artery & vein - Cervical lymph nodes	- Pressure on brachial plexus can cause paresthesia in upper extremity.
Deltopectoral triangle	Boundaries: - Medial 1/3 fibers of anterior Deltoid - Clavicle - Lateral 1/3 fibers of clavicular head of Pectoralis Major	- Brachial plexus - Axillary artery - Axillary vein - Subclavian vein - Cephalic vein - Deltoid branch of thoracoacromial artery	- Strong pressure directly inferior to coracoid process could compress the subclavian vein and axillary artery. - Working deeply under the clavicle could impinge the neurovascular bundle there.
Axillary region	Boundaries: - Anterior: Deltoid, Pectoralis Major - Posterior: Deltoid, Triceps, Latissimus Dorsi	- Axillary nerve, artery, vein, lymph nodes - Cephalic vein - Brachial plexus - Brachial artery	- Pectoralis Major, Pectoralis Minor and Subscapularis can be addressed well from the axillary area. Know how to navigate the anatomy before working here.

Endangerment Sites (continued)

Area of Concern	Location and Description	Endangered Structures	Comments
Medial brachium	- Space between adjacent borders of Biceps and Triceps Brachii	- Musculocutaneous nerve - Median nerve - Brachial artery - Basilic, brachial & cephalic veins - Radial nerve	- Know how to navigate the structures to avoid impinging the nerves and vessels.
Lateral epicondyle of humerus	Posterior elbow: - Proximal lateral epicondyle - Space between lateral epicondyle & olecranon process	- Radial nerve and its local branches	- A branch of the radial nerve courses just lateral to the tendon of Triceps Brachii. - Inflammation of this area is commonly known as "tennis elbow."
Medial epicondyle of humerus	Posterior elbow: - Area just proximal to medial epicondyle - Space between medial epicondyle & olecranon process	- Ulnar nerve - Ulnar artery	- Commonly known as the "funny bone." - Angle of elbow joint may affect the vulnerability of ulnar nerve. - Inflammation of this area is commonly known as "golfer's elbow."
Antecubital fossa	- Soft depression at the anterior elbow between common extensor tendon and common flexor tendon	- Median nerve - Radial nerve - Basilic vein - Brachial artery - Radial artery	- Caution when using cross-fiber friction on insertions of the Biceps Brachii & Brachialis in the shortened position because it may entrap the median nerve.
Xyphoid process	- Bony prominence at the inferior edge of sternum	- Xyphoid process	- Excessive pressure could damage bone
Abdominal region	- Soft area between the anterior rib cage and the pubic bone	- Liver, spleen, gallbladder, stomach, reproductive organs, intestines - Abdominal aorta - Vena cava - Vagus nerve	- If a pulse is palpated, you are on or near an artery, so redirect your contact. - Know how to navigate the territory and observe caution when applying manipulation to the viscera.

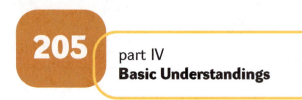

Endangerment Sites (continued)

Area of Concern	Location and Description	Endangered Structures	Comments
Low back region	- Level of upper lumbar vertebrae, just inferior to 12th rib	- Kidneys	- Strong and/or excessive percussive striking to the area may cause insult to the kidneys.
Sciatic notch	- Notch in pelvis between sacrum and greater trochanter	- Sciatic nerve	- When working Piriformis, be alert for referred pain.
Femoral triangle (also known as the inguinal triangle)	- Area bordered by Sartorius, inguinal ligament and Adductor Longus	- Femoral nerve - Femoral artery - Femoral vein - Great saphenous vein - Inguinal lymph nodes	- If a pulse is palpated, redirect your contact. - Be aware of the possibility of inguinal herniation.
Popliteal area	- Posterior knee between hamstrings above and Gastrocnemius below	- Tibial nerve (originates from sciatic nerve) - Popliteal artery - Popliteal nerve	- When working the posterior calf, take caution at medial head of fibula.

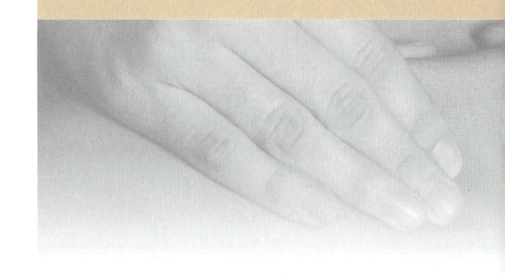

chapter 20

Practice Errors

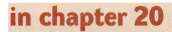

Practice Errors

Introduction

Some feel that no harm can result from a *BodyWork* session, that it just makes you feel good. Is that correct? Responsible practitioners know otherwise. They know that it is imperative to be knowledgeable regarding the structures they will contact and the impact their style of work will have upon these structures. They know that they must develop their *skills* and apply them in a safe manner to avoid negatively affecting their clients and themselves.

The overarching conversation related to safety issues is referred to as "medical errors." Because *BodyWorkers* don't practice medicine, a more appropriate term is "practice errors." To appreciate the primary concerns, it is best to understand some terms that reflect the issues.

Errors

An *error* is an occurrence that is viewed as problematic. It, most fundamentally, is an "oops." This can be an error of execution, meaning a failure of a planned action to be completed as intended ("I knew what to do, but I didn't manage to do it," or "I should have known but I forgot or neglected to utilize some *skill* or knowledge.") It can be an error of thought or planning, that is, the use of a wrong plan to achieve an aim (I misjudged the case and selected the wrong approach). It might also be an error of equipment where, due to poor quality, inferior maintenance or unskilled usage, a problem occurs. Fortunately, most *errors* do not result in serious consequences. Some never come to the attention of the therapist; others are noticed and then soon forgotten.

Adverse Events

An *adverse event*, however, is one where there is harm or injury to the client, an "oops" that goes bad. It is defined as an injury or death resulting from health care management, not from the underlying condition of the patient.

Malpractice

Malpractice is defined as the act or failure to act by a member of the health care profession that results in harm, injury, distress, prolonged physical or mental suffering or death. The practitioner, employer and/or product manufacturer may be held liable in cases that are litigated. The standard basis for determining *malpractice* is to compare the facts of the case to "the conduct of a reasonable, *skilled*, competent and experienced person who is a qualified member of the group authorized to engage in that professional activity."

Scope of Practice

Scope of practice refers to the range of activities included in a given profession. They may be determined by legislation (that which you are allowed to do by law), education (that for which you have adequate training), interest (that which you enjoy doing) and *skill* development (that which you are proficient in doing). Other influences would be a practitioner's size, endurance, life experiences, etc. A responsible practitioner respects and honors his/her personal *scope of practice* as determined by the above influences and refers out to others that which is determined to be beyond this scope.

History

The issue of *errors* in the practice of health care has been in the spotlight since the 1990s. This was mostly fueled by *iatrogenic* conditions in the practice of medicine such as when the wrong medication or the wrong dosage was administered to a patient, the wrong area of the *body* was operated on, a diagnosis was applied to the wrong patient or something was left in the *body* after an operation was complete. Early studies determined that as many as 98,000 deaths per year, the 8th leading cause of death at the time, were due to medical *errors* at a cost of $8.8 billion! Much progress and success has been achieved since then. Media articles have raised public awareness; health care systems scrutinized their procedures to better understand the problems and strategize solutions; and government agencies passed legislation to help reduce the occurrence of such tragedies.

During the early years of addressing problems related to practice *errors*, the focus was on *adverse events* in order to learn about the problems and strategize solutions. This directed the first wave of results-oriented responses. Now, researchers are also looking at "close calls" or "near misses" to better understand the systems, equipment, settings and procedures so as to establish guidelines that will even further reduce the occurrence of *errors* and *adverse events*.

"Issues of identifying and reducing health care error have drawn increasing attention in recent years. Many researchers and analysts advocate a move away from traditional approaches to health care error, which focus on individual responsibility and fault-finding, to an approach that stresses identification and correction of systems problems that lead to error."

Nursing World/Nursing Trends and Issues,
Vol. 3, No. 8, August 1998
www.nursingworld.org

A key aspect of a client safety environment is a culture that encourages practitioners, clients and others to be vigilant toward:

1. Identifying potential or actual errors
2. Taking appropriate steps to prevent and mitigate harm
3. Disclosing appropriate information on errors that do occur to facilitate learning

Errors in BodyWork

So, what are the *errors* related to BodyWork? They include failure to determine and respond to *contraindications*, failure to respect *endangerment sites*, overlooking or disregarding signals from the client, improper care of equipment and working with lubricants that have gone rancid or ones to which a client is sensitive. It is imperative that practitioners know the potential for harm inherent in their choice of *modality* and in their work environment.

Avoiding Errors

What might a therapist do to avoid *errors* and *adverse events*? First of all, **empower the client**. Let him or her know the options, the risks and the consequences of the work that will be done. A well-informed client can participate in choices from setting the goals for the session to selecting the *modality* to use. Their input may influence the timing and placement of applications. For instance, you may decide that the issues a client presents will be well served by deep tissue *techniques*. You inform him that the next day there may be residual discomfort from this work. He responds that he is engaging in a demanding physical activity the next day that would be challenging if he were in discomfort. Together, you

Factors and situations that increase the risk of errors:

- Fatigue
- Illness
- Inattention or distraction
- Emotional states
- Unfamiliar situations or problems
- Equipment design flaws
- Failure to maintain equipment in a safe, workable condition
- Inadequate labels or instructions on products or equipment
- Communication problems
- Unsafe working conditions

decide to postpone the deeper work for the next visit and that today's session will focus more on *general* relaxation.

Another step in preventing practice *errors* is **to take a client history and maintain session notes** in a way that is appropriate to your practice. This requires knowing the potential issues related to your work. The specific information you need from an athlete will differ somewhat from what you want to know about an elderly person. The information you need when performing Structural Integration will differ from what you need for a Polarity session. This history can be very general or highly specific in relation to your specialty. It can be verbal or written. Depending on your setting and the work you do, a written history may be preferable. Jotting some notes afterward about the session may serve as a valuable reference. When communicating with doctors, insurance companies or lawyers in relation to a client, you would need to have written documentation to submit or refer to. In settings where written histories are not taken, at least verbally ask for the particular information needed.

Apply your **knowledge of indications and contraindications** as related to your practice. A condition that *contraindicates* one type of response may *indicate* another.

Know your anatomy and physiology as appropriate to your practice. You don't have to remember every little detail, but know when, where and how to reference the necessary information. Establish your own or have access to a good resource library and charts related to your work.

Be present with your clients and attentive to the information that you gather from the intake process. Keep lines of communication open between you and your clients, i.e., encourage feedback and check in with them throughout the session.

Look for response signals such as facial expressions, flinching, resistance, or *local* erythema that would suggest caution or adjusting your focus or *technique*.

"...To make health care safe we need to redesign our systems to make errors difficult to commit, and create a culture in which the existence of risk is acknowledged and injury prevention is recognized as everyone's responsibility."

Lucien Leape, 1998, www.nursingceu.com, pg. 11

"When the number one killer in a society is the healthcare system, then, that system has no excuse except to address its own urgent shortcomings. It's a failed system in need of immediate attention."

Gary Null, PhD,
Carolyn Dean, MD, ND,
Martin Feldman, MD,
Debora Rasio, MD,
Death by Medicine - 8,
November 2003,
www.garynull.com

Maintain your equipment and ensure that you are properly trained to use it. This means, regularly check that the nuts and bolts holding your table together are tight, that any cables or wires are not fraying and that moving parts are lubricated. Make sure that electrical equipment is calibrated correctly and that wires and plugs are intact. Ensure that you are trained and confident in your knowledge and *skill* to use the equipment.

Know and respect the range and limitations of your knowledge and *skills*, that is, honestly **identify your "personal" scope of practice**. If you want to broaden your scope, go to the best source you can to get additional training. Maintain and update your *skills* and knowledge through self-study and continuing education. Stay abreast of the latest information available by reading professional journals, networking with others and taking at least one seminar or workshop a year. This not only keeps you current, it also keeps you engaged and expands your *skills* so that you stay jazzed and excited about doing *BodyWork*.

What should you do if you discover an error? Ask three questions:
1. What happened?
2. Why did it happen?
3. What can be done to prevent it from happening again?

The answers to these questions will inform and direct any changes, additions or corrections to your existing practices and procedures. Remember, to avoid practice errors, client safety is paramount when organizing your workspace, designing your overall systems and implementing your practice.

Tips to avoid practice errors:

- Empower the client

- Take a client history

- Maintain session notes

- Check for contraindications

- Know anatomy and physiology

- Be present with your clients

- Look for response signals

- Maintain your equipment

- Stay within your personal scope of practice

part

V

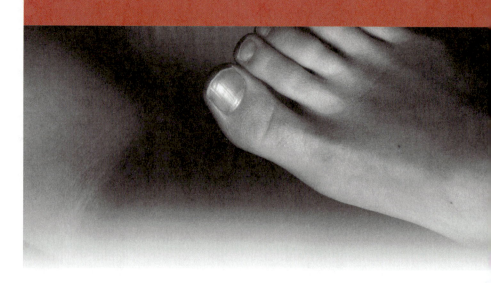

Becoming an Integrated BodyWorker

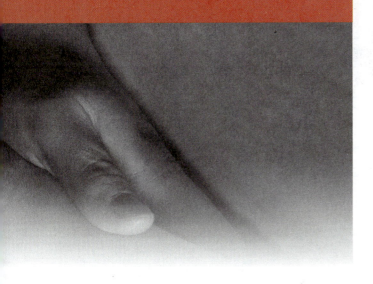

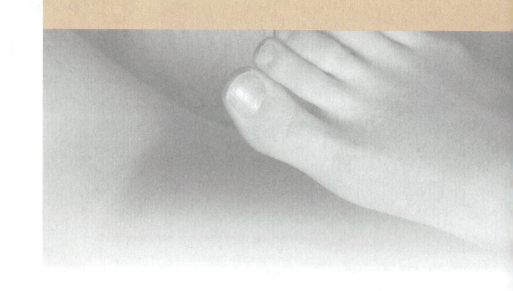

chapter 21

Putting It All Into Practice

Putting It All Into Practice

Introduction

Touch is a nonverbal language of communication. It is an outlet for emotional expression. We can express pleasure or displeasure, joy or sadness, good or ill will. As *BodyWork* practitioners, we gather as large a vocabulary of touch *skills* as we can to serve our own and our clients' highest good.

Options

As you are exposed to various *techniques* and philosophies, keep in mind that there are a vast number of possible ways to connect. Each possibility represents a physical and energetic option for one human *body* to interact with another. Such interactions might include *skills* such as pressing, rubbing, squeezing, stroking, sensing, visualizing and pacing among others. The variety of applications becomes limitless when we combine *skills* and weave them with various qualities of touch and a multitude of intentions.

In working with a client, assess the person's needs, then choose from your acquired *skills* to create in that moment, a session (or series of sessions) for that particular situation. When working consistently with a certain population or with a specific intention or purpose you might discover repeatable combinations of *skills* that support desired outcomes.

Study

Exposure to a wide variety of thinkers in the ways of touch is important. Be open to hear their philosophy, how they view the *body* in function and dysfunction, how they experience the role they play in supporting a person to greater health, and how they express this through their particular approach.

Each *modality* that you come across may have a piece that can be incorporated into your own emerging practice. If you are attracted to, and resonate with, a certain philosophy or approach, learn it as fully as you can from as rich a source as you can find.

Exploration

Always stay open to whatever might enhance your work. It is good to maintain a playful heart and inquisitive mind because some of your greatest discoveries occur when you are just exploring. Give yourself permission to discover new territory, innovative *techniques*, and deeper understandings of the subtle relationships that can occur between client and therapist.

You may find that others will lay claim to discovering the same things you have. This is not only possible, but commonplace. Enjoy the personal power of your discovery as you uncover the mysteries that are available to all who seek them. It is exciting and rewarding. Your clients will be forever grateful.

Creative Expression

Allow yourself free and creative expression as you expand your own repertoire of touch *skills*. It is our personal belief that there is no room for limiting dogma in health care. Just look for and use what works!   It is also important to recognize and honor your limits regarding your *skills* and training. If a situation suggests an approach that is outside your realm of expertise, it is best to refer out to a practitioner who can competently provide the needed service.

Integrity

A weekend workshop, or short introductory class rarely makes you an expert. Do not fool yourself or those who come to you by misrepresenting your *skills*. This doesn't mean you should not practice what you have just learned, just let your clients know the truth. Unless you are fully trained and proficient, as well as certified or licensed in a particular *technique* or approach (where such a thing is available), do not include this in your advertising or promote yourself as such. For example, if you have only taken an introductory course in Shiatsu, do not advertise or say on your business card that you do Shiatsu. Tell your clients that you have taken a short course, but do not suggest you are an expert.

"There is a natural progression in manual therapy from the gross to the subtle, from the fascial matrix to the energy matrix, from working on someone to working with someone, from overcoming resistance to establishing trust. As one learns to listen...a whole new world of subtle rhythms and forces is revealed."

Tom McDonough
Massage Magazine
May/June 1998,
No. 73, pg.93

"Connection and bonding have to do with how experience gets organized, how it is transferred to others, and how it is interjected to become a part of one's self...the main tools a therapist has are his own responses...how he responds to what this person evokes in him and to understand his place in dealing with the client– that is what needs to be addressed. A therapeutic process is not objective. Even if a therapist keeps a distance, it is still a personal relationship."

Stanley Keleman,
Bonding, 1986

"Most people don't realize that education is not the event of me teaching you, it is the process of your taking initiative for learning. The teacher, the school is just a resource. The teacher's role is to motivate and guide. The student's role is to search and investigate, and to thereby discover truth and knowledge for themselves.... The word 'doctor' means 'teacher,' and whether teaching in a classroom or a treatment room, the essential purpose and focus is the same: to uplift the human spirit through truth. Truth about our health, and truth about our purpose in life, as massage therapists and as healers."

Ralph Stephens,
Massage Today,
September 2002,
Vol. 2, No. 9, pg. 8

Integration

If you begin a new course of study after you have become well practiced and proficient in one approach, you may experience your work as less fluid than before. Do not be discouraged, as the initial phase of learning new *skills* often feels cerebral and mechanical. This is just a stage in which the nervous system is being retrained with different patterns of behavior. As time and practice will show, these *skills* will become integrated with previously learned ones and your work will once again become fluid and intuitive.

Begin with a sensitive heart and an open mind. Maintain this openness and the world will continue to feel fresh with new possibilities. We ripen with experience. In the *field* of *BodyWork*, learning never ends. Enjoy the journey!

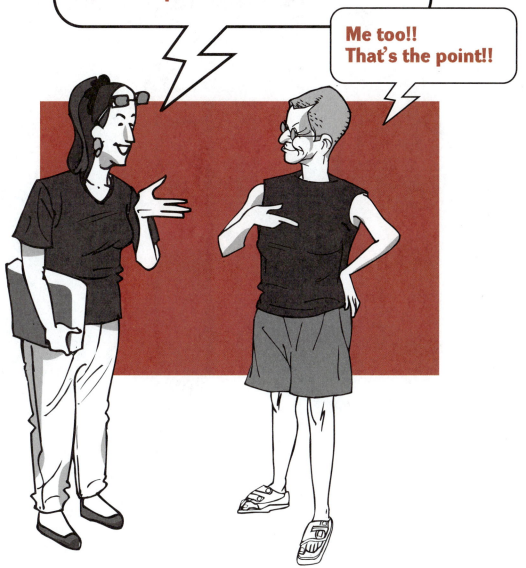

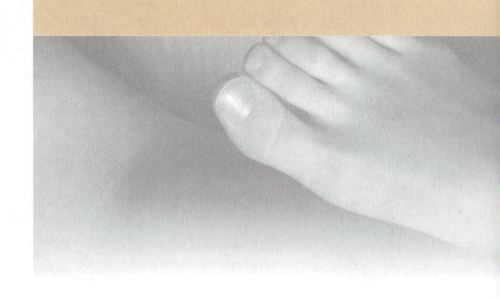

chapter **22**

Attaining Mastery

Attaining Mastery

Introduction

The one thing in the world that is absolutely constant is change. It is ongoing and endless. The streaming of life-force energy that animates everything is reflected in the ever-shifting and emerging *body*. Effective *BodyWork* is a flow of instantaneous responses to this dynamic of perpetual change. It begins with a therapist who is sensitive to the signals of the *body* and *skilled* in the ways of touch and connection. It calls for *mastery*.

Mastery Defined

What is *mastery*? It is competence, proficiency, the possession of profound knowledge. It is a combination of *skill*, wisdom and expertise. It is the level of excellence that sets one therapist apart from another. *Mastery* manifests as a high-level integration of *skill*, focus and strategy.

The Whole Client

When we play with another *body* we are playing with the active principle in that person's *body*—how they hold themselves, their life force, how they move, what traumas, what emotions and what ideas they embody. We are interacting with something that is alive, which is dynamic and part of the great mystery. A person is an energetic *field* of action potential, time frames and history. Their biography shows up in their biology. When we touch somebody, this is what we are touching.

Developing Wisdom

Certain things can be taught and others can only be learned. That's why touching the first thousand *bodies* is so important. It provides a series of introductions to subtle signs that collect in your inner experience that make sense when you have accumulated enough of them. *Mastery* is not acquired intellectually; it is attained experientially in increments that emerge collectively to become wisdom and intelligence.

Touch *skills* are not just conceptual; they are stimulated and developed through practice. *Techniques* are the medium for developing these *skills*; practice refines them with precision and knowing, yet practice alone is not always enough to keep you excited and at your edge.

Supporting Mastery

What supports *mastery*? What advances competency and expertise and inspires optimal performance?

- Continuing education seminars
- Trades with fellow therapists
- Reading the latest books and professional journals
- Networking with other practitioners
- Participating in professional associations
- Receiving coaching from more advanced practitioners

For the most part, *BodyWork* is a singular experience. The one-on-one nature of a session does not provide the practitioner with peer interaction and stimulation. Just think of the benefit one could gain from connecting to others who do the same thing. Imagine the support available by networking at a professional organization meeting, interacting with fellow students at a continuing education seminar or trading *BodyWork* with other therapists. There is power in joining a study group, reading the latest publications or mentoring someone else to grow as a therapist.

Coaching and Mentoring

Connecting with a personal coach or mentor can provide more focused, individualized assistance and encouragement. A coach or mentor is a trusted seasoned guide who can offer another perspective and serve as a mirror for self-examination. They can confirm experiences practitioners have with their work or provide feedback, direction, inspiration, guidance and objective input that deepens understanding and stimulates new perceptions and connections.

Masterful *BodyWork* is more than just the key ingredients and fundamental elements of a *technique*, *skill* or approach being used. Ultimately it is about training, *presence*, practice, preparation, perception and the ability to move beyond what you already know.

"Mentors and apprentices are partners in an ancient human dance, and one of teaching's great rewards is the daily chance it gives us to get back on the dance floor. It is the dance of the spiraling generations, in which the old empower the young with their experience and the young empower the old with new life, reweaving the fabric of the human community as they touch and turn."

Parker J. Palmer, The Courage to Teach: Exploring the Inner Landscape of a Teacher's Life, 1998

"Ultimately, a person who seeks training in BodyWork is answering a calling to a meaningful vocation.... The second half of the journey is to establish a meaningful self identity. Thus transpersonal education affirms the value and correctness of subjective experience and places a great value on self-actualization.... All the teacher can really do is facilitate a learning situation. The focus of transpersonal education is not on the material the teacher presents, but on what the student discovers within himself or herself."

Michael Shea, The Art of Teaching Touch: Theory and Practice of Adult Learning and Development, 1998

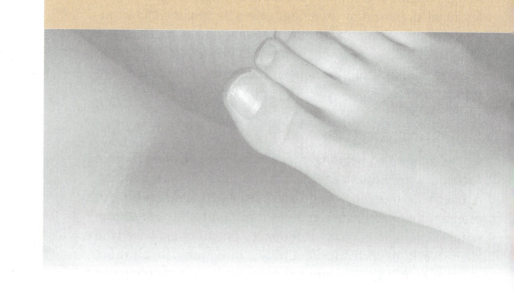

chapter **23**

Linking TouchAbilities® to Modalities

Linking TouchAbilities® to Modalities

Introduction

We celebrate *modalities*! Because there are so many of them we have variety, options, choices, growth and moment-to-moment uniqueness of experience. All the different approaches bring us different dances, different *rhythms*, different moods, different textures, different options.

What Is a Modality?

So what is a *modality*? Fundamentally, a *modality* is a selection of *techniques* compiled and organized to meet a challenge. It is a system based on a specific view of, and guided by a particular philosophy regarding the *body*. *Technique* alone does not a *modality* make. The unique nature of any approach is determined by the *BodyView*, the qualities of touch, the selection and combination of touch *skills* and the underlying intention of the work.

Who Creates a Modality?

Who creates a *modality*? It could be anyone. What do you think happened for Ida Rolf, Moshe Feldenkrais or Randolph Stone? They were facing challenges that could not be met by the current practices of the time. Imagine you, or someone you know, are facing a challenge. You search for someone or something that can help. Nothing you find seems to work. You start to experiment and figure things out for yourself. Through creativity and observation, through trial and error, you discover ways that consistently make improvements. You share your discoveries with others who face similar situations and someone asks you to teach your approach. Before you know it, therapists practice it; clients seek it out. Congratulations! You're the "someone" who has created a new *modality*.

Primordial Soup

This chapter is about such creation. It is about lineage, linkage and opening your mind to a broad range of possibilities. When we started, we thought we'd distill the essence of each approach and make a universal chart with a general explanation. In the process, we noticed a variation among practitioners' responses, even people within the same *modality*. Each system has unifying ideas and principles and then there are the human factors of interpretation and practice. In some instances we just had to include more than one version of the same *modality* to demonstrate this point. On the surface, all *modalities* appear different, one from the other. However, once the subject is peeled down through the layers to its core actions, no matter what the system calls them, we see that everyone is dipping into the same primordial soup of *skills*.

Charts

On the following pages we identify a variety of *modalities* that are representative of approaches available today. We invited many practitioners and primary teachers in the field to contribute to this chapter. These contributors distinguish the basic concepts and list the *techniques* or intentions most commonly utilized by them within a given *modality*. Then, each technique is directly correlated to its source *skill/s* from TouchAbilities®. As you study these charts it will become obvious to you how TouchAbilities® is universally represented in the *skillset* of, and serves as the fundamental basis for, the wide range of *modalities* already in existence and foundational for those yet to be created.

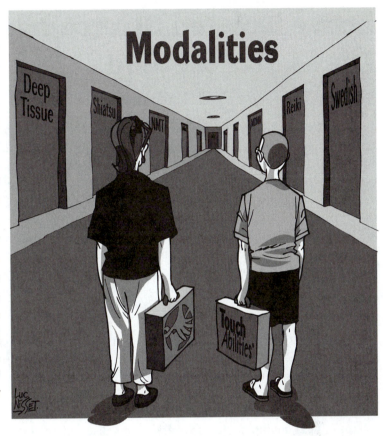

Many *modalities* focus strictly on the physical, biomechanical plane and don't include the intangible aspects of the *body*. Some are more strongly rooted in the subtle realms and feature specific *techniques* and intentions designed to play only in these *domains*. Then there are *modalities* that are all-encompassing.

Eclecticism

The trend today is toward integration and eclecticism. As you read this chapter on *modalities*, make distinctions and look for commonalities, differences and crossovers among them. It is empowering to study a *modality* in depth to get its essence, value and potential. Magic happens when you take new options and blend them with whatever you are already doing. When they integrate into your *body*, they become part of your repertoire, your *skillset*, and are readily available as you work with a client in a given moment.

Different moves open different doorways. Different moves open the same doorways. Coming from a TouchAbilities® background makes learning a new *modality* as easy as walking through a different doorway. Follow your heart and learn all you can.

Active Isolated Stretching: The Mattes Method

Aaron Mattes

Aaron Mattes' Active Isolated Stretching (AIS) method of fascial release provides effective dynamic facilitated stretch of major muscle groups. This leads to functional and physiological restoration of superficial and deep fascial planes. Performing an Active Isolated Stretch of no greater than 2.0 seconds allows the target muscle(s) to optimally lengthen without triggering the protective stretch reflex and subsequent reciprocal antagonist muscle contraction.

AIS *techniques* are applied in two phases. Phase I, *Assisted Active Isolated Stretching*, is characterized by the client's focused mental concentration throughout the action. The therapist directs the client in a given movement and assists by applying less than one pound of pressure to help increase tissue and joint range. The improvement in body realignment, pain relief, energy, ambulatory capacity, athletic potential and rehabilitation is rapidly accomplished.

During phase II, *Active Isolated Stretching*, the client is taught to use reciprocal innervation and inhibition to achieve the desired result. This helps clients to maintain improvements, increase self-awareness and assume responsibility for their health status.

Clients presenting with spinal cord injury, neurological deficits of varying nature, amyotrophic lateral sclerosis (ALS), multiple sclerosis, Parkinson's disease, head trauma, spinal distortions, foot distortions and orthopedic problems all respond well to AIS. It is used with everyone from preschool children to professional athletes. Psychiatric patients with various mental and emotional problems are being treated with AIS and prison systems are now experimenting with how AIS might affect deep-seated hatred or aggressive behavior.

AIS very specifically uses precise movements of short duration (2.0 seconds) and minimum force of under 1 pound of assistive pressure. This method is consistently successful in the treatment of deep and long-standing pain. It is a valuable tool that is often integrated into the work of other *BodyWork* professionals.

Active Isolated Stretching

TouchAbilities®

Technique	Component	Skill
*See paragraph below	Kinetics	Holding, Supporting, Mobilizing, Stabilizing
	Expansion	Pulling, Lifting
	Breathing	Tracking, Directing, Pacing
	Cognitive	Visualizing, Inquiring, Intending, Focusing, Transmitting
	Energetic	Sensing, Intuiting, Balancing

* Active Isolated Stretching and Assisted Active Isolated Stretching utilize the following therapeutic intentions:

- Identifying the muscles to be stretched
- Isolating the muscles to be stretched by using precise *localized* movements
- Intensifying the contractile effort of the agonist muscle/s to enhance relaxation and lengthening of the antagonist muscle/s on the opposite side of the joint
- Repeating isotonic contractions to increase *local* blood flow, oxygen and nutrition; and move lymph, enhancing *local* physiological well-being

These intentions are accomplished by employing various combinations of the above TouchAbilities® *skills* as needed in the moment.

The Benjamin System of Muscular Therapy

Ben Benjamin

The Benjamin System of Muscular Therapy was developed by Ben Benjamin from a synthesis of several approaches to working with the body. Benjamin designed a series of muscular manipulations based on the work of Alfred Kagan, who developed original *techniques* for the treatment of muscular tension and injury. Benjamin also incorporates ideas from Dr. Wilhelm Reich on the emotional *component* of muscular tension; from F. M. Alexander on the relationship of faulty movement habits to pain, tension and injury; and from Dr. James Cyriax on injury *assessment* and friction therapy.

Muscular Therapy treatments include *massage*, using area-specific *techniques* and a variety of pressures, speeds and *rhythms* to reduce *chronic* tension and pain; client education about the causes and effects of tension; and client self-care *techniques* to prevent the build-up of new tension. Benjamin's Orthopedic Massage: Injury Assessment and Treatment includes a series of specific *assessments* to determine the precise location of injuries, friction treatment to muscles, tendons and ligaments, *massage*, and exercises to promote tissue healing and strength.

Muscular Therapy *techniques* consist of using portions of the hand and arm (palmar surface, finger pads, knuckles, pisiform bone, ulnar surface, elbow, etc.) to apply varying pressures at varying speeds to specific muscles and muscle groups; applying tractions and holds; moving, rocking, shaking or compressing areas of the body; and applying cross-fiber friction to tendons and ligaments. Depending on the particular *technique* selected, the intent may be to manually lengthen and separate muscle fibers, increase the space in joint capsules, use the neuromuscular system to stimulate relaxation, increase the depth of respiration, or break down scar tissue. Each Muscular Therapy session is based on *assessment* of the client, constructed to address the individual needs of a client, and takes into consideration the physical, emotional and mental *state* of the client. Sessions are marked by collaboration between the client and therapist, clear boundaries and respect for each individual.

Benjamin System of Muscular Therapy

TouchAbilities®

Technique	Component	Skill
*See paragraph below	Breathing	Tracking, Directing, Pacing
	Cognitive	Inquiring, Intending, Focusing, Transmitting
	Energetic	Sensing, Intuiting, Balancing
	Compression	Pressing/Pushing, Squeezing/Pinching, Twisting
	Expansion	Pulling, Lifting, Rolling
	Kinetic	Holding/Supporting, Mobilizing, Stabilizing
	Oscillation	Vibrating, Shaking
	Gliding	Sliding, Planing, Rubbing

* Benjamin System of Muscular Therapy *techniques* are not segmented and named in a linear manner. What is taught are intentions, and the methods to achieve those intentions. There is also a specific focus on developing efficient *body mechanics*. The *techniques* employed by the Benjamin System may be correlated to the above TouchAbilities® Components and *skills*.

Bhakti Energy Work™

Julie and Dale McNitt

Bhakti Energy Work™ is a metamodel of *BodyWork*. The intent of this work is consciousness. Consciousness is energy, mind and body. Inspired by the teachings of Eckhart Tolle and <u>A Course in Miracles</u>, the core belief of Bhakti is that "cause and effect are one." The goal is to become conscious and respond with *presence* in the moment.

So that they can be in the present moment, Bhakti Energy Work™ supports individuals to fully experience what they feel, facilitating them to clear out their internal environment of past feelings/emotions/energies. Bhakti Energy Work™ can be experienced on a Somatron Mat™ (a music source is imbedded in the mat), a *BodyWork* table, a floor mat or in the water. It can also be experienced sitting, standing, or from a distance, as in distance healing. This work focuses on meridians, chakras, and includes sweeps on and off the body.

Bhakti Energy Work™ is a meditative dance, which is often described as a spiritual awakening. It focuses on four **Constants: Constant Attention** (the ultimate goal), **Constant Movement**, **Constant Pace** and **Constant Pressure**. The work flows harmoniously from one part of the body to another and the pace, compared to most styles, is extremely slow. A long gliding stroke could likely take 3 minutes or as long as 30 minutes to go from the foot up the leg and back and down the arm to the hand. A Bhakti session has a hypnotic effect and the slow strokes allow the client to move into deep levels of relaxation, and even altered *states*.

All of Bhakti Energy Work™ is about becoming conscious. Only a conscious person has a choice. Healing is about bringing us closer to consciousness. Cure, which is the absence of symptoms, may or may not follow. Awareness of one's intent, breath, and senses, along with visualizations are all part of the process. This therapy is designed to help both client and practitioner connect with their own internal guidance. The goal is to have them develop trust in themselves and look to themselves, the present moment and discover what IS.

Bhakti Energy Work™   TouchAbilities®

Technique	Component	Skill
Establishing Presence	Breathing	Tracking, Directing, Pacing
	Cognitive	Visualizing, Inquiring, Intending, Focusing
Holding Intention	Energetic	Sensing, Intuiting, Balancing
Developing Consciousness	Gliding	Sliding, Rubbing

All other TouchAbilities® *techniques* may be incorporated as the needs of the moment dictate. Because the essence of Bhakti Energy Work™ is **presence** and **consciousness**, it allows for any form of physical or energetic connection to manifest. This system does not specify particular *techniques*. Rather, practitioners direct an intention and remain open for any *technique* to come forward intuitively as needed in the moment. This would naturally include any and all of the TouchAbilities® elements. Therefore, a chart for this *modality* would be one that mimics the entire TouchAbilities® chart with a very strong emphasis on the *techniques* within the Breathing, Cognitive, Energetic and Gliding Components.

Chair Massage – TouchPro®

David Palmer

TouchPro® Chair Massage, created by David Palmer, is derived from a traditional form of Japanese table *massage* and the theoretical foundations of Traditional Chinese Medicine (TCM) which recognizes the interaction of body/mind/spirit. The functional intention of the work is to enhance circulation so that the client's body can heal itself.

Sitting in a specially designed *massage* chair opens up the back muscles, relieves strain on the neck and provides gentle relief for the eyes. Chair Massage supports *homeostatic* balance by keeping little problems from escalating into big ones. An average of 15 minutes on the neck, back, arms and hands can increase circulation, improve energy levels and protect against injury.

Whether caused by stress, sitting behind a desk or standing all day, shopping or traveling, tight muscles can impede blood and lymph flow. The result could be fatigue, mental fogginess and decreased energy. Chair Massage counters the circulatory problems inherent with these *stressors*.

The TouchPro® system provides a specific form and sequence to follow to achieve definitive results. Therapists perform anywhere from 5 to 30 minute *massages* on seated clients. This approach is designed to be efficient for practitioners of all shapes and sizes and effective at promoting relaxation and circulation for a broad spectrum of clients no matter what their size, age, level of wellness and/or touch history.

Chair Massage is practiced in a variety of locations from shopping malls and airports to corporate workplaces and community events. There is no remedial or medical intention behind the TouchPro® approach. The client does not get undressed, it is not necessary to use lubricants and it can be administered in a public place. In this way, it offers a comfortable, nonthreatening environment for someone to open to the benefits of touch. This simple relaxation protocol can be used to educate people about *BodyWork* as well as develop a client base for table work.

TouchPro®

TouchAbilities®

Technique	Component	Skill
Client Screening	Cognitive	Inquiring, Intending
Palm Press	Compression	Pressing
Archer's Arm	Compression	Pressing
Forearm Press	Compression	Pressing
Elbow Press	Compression	Pressing
Duckbill Squeeze	Compression	Squeezing
Thumb Press	Compression	Pressing
Spreading the Hands	Gliding	Sliding, Rubbing
Stroke & Jiggle	Gliding	Sliding, Rubbing
Coin Rub	Gliding	Planing, Rubbing
Arm Stretch	Expansion Oscillation	Pulling Vibrating
Neck Stretch	Kinetic	Mobilizing
Chicken Wing Stretch	Kinetic	Mobilizing
Angel Wing Stretch	Kinetic	Mobilizing
Hip Rotations	Gliding	Sliding, Rubbing
Ten-finger Scalp Massage	Gliding Compression	Planing Pressing
Crab Grab	Expansion	Pulling, Lifting
Thumb Squeeze Rotations	Compression	Pressing, Twisting

TouchPro®
(continued)

TouchAbilities®

Technique	Component	Skill
Waterfall Brush	Gliding	Sliding
Shoulder Drops	Kinetic	Letting Go/Dropping
Loose Fist Percussion	Oscillation	Striking
Praying Hands Percussion	Oscillation	Striking
Cupped Hands Percussion	Oscillation	Striking

CORE Somatic BodyWork
Structural Integration & Myofascial Therapy

George Kousaleos

CORE Somatic BodyWork is rooted in Ida Rolf's Structural Integration. CORE Structural Therapy follows the 10-session "recipe" and includes flexibility and awareness exercises that increase the client's potential for neurosomatic awareness. Each session works on progressively deeper layers of *fascia*, musculature and ligaments to provide improved structural alignment and functional abilities. CORE Myofascial Therapy is a moderate full-body system that uses the basic *techniques* of structural integration to release the superficial tension of outer layers of both *fascia* and musculature. It has been successfully used as a training therapy for athletes, dancers and other performers. The study and practice of CORE Myofascial Therapy is a prerequisite for learning CORE Structural Integration.

CORE Somatic BodyWork utilizes an understanding of the important roles that *fascia* and myofascia, both dense fibrous connective tissues, have in the human body. Not only are they a strong and resilient soft-tissue that surrounds, supports and guides all musculoskeletal movement, the outermost layer of *fascia* also provides a framework for the lymphatic, venous return and sensory nervous systems.

CORE therapists use the leverage of their whole body to apply pressure at a 45-degree angle to the anterior, posterior and both lateral planes of the body. Utilizing their palms, fingers, fist, knuckles, forearms and elbows, CORE therapists apply a bilateral pressure along the grain of *fascia*. The success of these *techniques* is based on a slow application of pressure, allowing the client to relax more deeply with each stroke. The goal of all the *techniques* is to "create space" in the soft-tissues, allowing for more effortless movement.

For clients to maintain the structural benefits of each session, they are taught a standing isometric exercise that gradually improves length, balance and awareness. Flexibility exercises for the neck, shoulders, back, hips and legs are also taught with sessions that focus on specific regions of the body.

Like all forms of structural integration, CORE Somatic Bodywork can increase the client's ability to process personal psychological issues. Indeed, the session work can bring to the surface repressed emotions from traumatic experiences. Understanding these physical/psychological relationships enables the client to enjoy a heightened *state* of mental and emotional balance.

CORE Somatic Bodywork

TouchAbilities®

Technique	Component	Skill
Myofascial Spreading/Stretching	Gliding	Planing
Broad Cross-Fiber Friction	Gliding	Rubbing
Digital Compression	Compression	Pressing
Broad Tissue Compression	Compression	Pushing
Traction	Expansion	Pulling
Joint Range of Motion	Kinetics	Mobilizing
Joint/Arthro Kinetics	Kinetics	Stabilizing
Client Assessment	Cognitive	Visualizing, Inquiring
Client Education	Cognitive	Transmitting, Intending
Breathing Awareness	Breathing	Tracking, Directing

Cranial Sacral Therapy

Avi-Khadir Aberman

Cranial Sacral Therapy is a gentle, noninvasive manual therapy that addresses the health and function of the central nervous system, the autonomic nervous system and the tissues that nourish and protect them. These tissues include the meninges of the central nervous system (CNS), the bones of the cranium, spine and sacrum, and the fluids that circulate within them. Because the nervous and endocrine systems help to regulate, repair and coordinate all the other systems and functions of the body/mind, this therapy affects a person on physical, emotional, mental and spiritual levels.

Osteopath William Sutherland originally discovered and described this system of "primary respiration" in which cerebrospinal fluid carries a subtle healing energy and distributes it throughout the body via pulsations of the fluid, bone, membrane and neural *components*. Cranial Sacral *techniques* can be grouped into two general categories. In the first, a therapist may apply gentle pressure to release restrictions, which frees motion through the sutures and permits the system to resume proper function.

Secondly, the therapist directs his/her attention into the system and becomes aware of the subtle energies and movements within it. No attempt is made to correct a problem. The body is approached in a manner that allows self-correction in the most exact and efficient way possible. The practitioner does not "do" anything, only maintains a *state* of awareness, which somehow allows the energy ("potency") of the system to make the necessary corrections.

Regardless of which *techniques* are applied, when the cranial sacral system functions more efficiently a wide range of remarkable effects occur. Almost always, pain is diminished and becomes less disturbing. The mind relaxes and becomes clear; emotional blocks may be released. Immune function is enhanced and there is improvement in the body's response to stress. Many people experience what they describe as greater spiritual clarity or a deep sense of being nourished from within. Some people report that old, unwanted life patterns dissolve away, leaving them better able to build more effective ones.

Cranial Sacral Therapy complements and synergistically increases the effectiveness of other *BodyWork modalities*. It needs no special tools or equipment, only a calm quiet space, and can be applied without removing clothes. Because it requires little or no physical force in application, individuals who do not possess the strength or physical endowment required for many other *modalities* can perform it effectively.

Cranial Sacral Therapy

TouchAbilities®

Technique	Component	Skill
Occipital "Cradle" Hold	Cognitive	Visualizing, Focusing, Transmitting, Inquiring, Intending
	Energetic	Sensing, Intuiting, Balancing
	Kinetic	Holding/Supporting, Stabilizing
Diaphragm Release	Cognitive	Visualizing, Focusing, Transmitting, Inquiring, Intending
	Energetic	Sensing, Intuiting, Balancing
	Compression	Pressing/Pushing, Twisting
	Expansion	Lifting, Pulling
	Kinetic	Holding/Supporting
CV4- Stillpoint Induction	Cognitive	Visualizing, Focusing, Transmitting, Inquiring, Intending
	Energetic	Sensing, Intuiting, Balancing
	Compression	Pressing/Pushing
	Kinetic	Holding/Supporting
Atlas-Occiput Release	Energetic	Sensing, Intuiting, Balancing
	Compression	Pressing/Pushing
	Expansion	Lifting, Pulling
	Kinetic	Holding/Supporting
Temporal "Ear Pull" Release	Cognitive	Visualizing, Focusing, Transmitting, Inquiring, Intending
	Energetic	Sensing, Intuiting, Balancing
	Compression	Twisting
	Expansion	Pulling
	Kinetic	Holding/Supporting

Cranial Sacral Therapy (continued)

TouchAbilities®

Technique	Component	Skill
Sacral "Cradle" Hold	Cognitive	Visualizing, Focusing, Transmitting, Inquiring, Intending
	Energetic	Sensing, Intuiting, Balancing
	Compression	Pressing/Pushing
	Expansion	Lifting, Pulling
	Kinetic	Holding/Supporting

CranioSacral Therapy

Sheryl McGavin (for John Upledger)

CranioSacral Therapy is a gentle, hands-on method of whole-body evaluation and care that can have a positive impact on every system of the body. It was developed by osteopathic physician John E. Upledger in the mid-1970s after years of university research and clinical testing.

CranioSacral Therapy helps normalize the craniosacral system, which consists of the membranes and cerebrospinal fluid that surround and protect the central nervous system, i.e., the brain, spinal cord and all related structures. Restrictions or imbalances in the craniosacral system may directly affect any or all aspects of central nervous system performance, which in turn can negatively affect the entire body. CranioSacral Therapy practitioners are trained to use gentle *palpation* to detect and address these problems by facilitating the inherent self-correcting abilities of the body.

Generally using about 5 grams of pressure, roughly the weight of a nickel, the CranioSacral Therapy practitioner palpates the *rhythmic* movement of cerebrospinal fluid circulating within the craniosacral system to assess the ease of motion and locate areas of restriction. This enables the practitioner to discover and work with the origin of the symptoms of the disease or dysfunction. Specific treatment *techniques* are then used to facilitate release of restrictions in fasciae, membranes and any other tissues that are found during the *assessment* to be influencing the craniosacral system. The result is an improved internal environment for the central nervous system allowing it to return to its optimal levels of health and performance.

The gentle touch used in CranioSacral Therapy is essential to work with the self-correcting abilities of the body– to facilitate rather than direct the treatment process. It enables the therapist to feel and respond to the subtle changes and movements that occur in the body when specific *techniques* are used and to gently initiate, follow and support release of restrictions. Because the body has no need to defend against this gentle, nondirective approach to treatment, there can often be significant, long lasting changes.

The focus on the origins of dysfunction and the gentle touch used have made CranioSacral Therapy an effective treatment approach for a wide variety of conditions. It has been found to be beneficial for brain and spinal cord injuries, migraines and headaches, chronic fatigue syndrome, motor-coordination impairments, neck and back pain, scoliosis, central nervous system disorders, emotional difficulties, temporomandibular joint (TMJ) syndrome, learning disabilities, stress and tension-related problems, post-traumatic stress disorder, orthopedic problems and many others.

CranioSacral Therapy

TouchAbilities®

Technique	Component	Skill
Whole-Body Assessment	Breathing	Tracking
	Cognitive	Focusing, Intending, Inquiring
	Energetic	Sensing
	Kinetic	Mobilizing
	Gliding	Sliding/Planing
Still Point Induction	Kinetic	Mobilizing, Letting Go, Holding/Supporting
	Cognitive	Focusing, Intending
	Energetic	Sensing
	Breathing	Tracking
Diaphragm Releases	Breathing	Tracking
	Cognitive	Focusing, Intending
	Energetic	Sensing
	Compression	Pressing/Pushing
	Expansion	Pulling
	Kinetic	Holding/Supporting, Letting Go, Stabilizing
	Gliding	Sliding/Planing
Direction of Energy	Cognitive	Intending, Focusing, Transmitting, Visualizing
	Energetic	Sensing
Intracranial Membrane Techniques	Cognitive	Intending, Focusing
	Energetic	Sensing
	Compression	Pressing/Pushing
	Expansion	Pulling
	Kinetic	Mobilizing, Letting Go, Holding/Supporting
	Gliding	Sliding/Planing

CranioSacral Therapy (continued)

TouchAbilities®

Technique	Component	Skill
Dural Tube Techniques	Cognitive	Intending, Focusing
	Energetic	Sensing
	Compression	Pressing/Pushing
	Expansion	Pulling
	Kinetic	Mobilizing, Letting Go, Holding/Supporting
	Gliding	Sliding/Planing
Positional Tissue Release	Cognitive	Intending, Focusing
	Breathing	Tracking
	Energetic	Sensing
	Compression	Pressing/Pushing
	Expansion	Pulling
	Kinetic	Mobilizing, Letting Go, Holding/Supporting
	Gliding	Sliding/Planing
SomatoEmotional Release®	Breathing	Tracking
	Cognitive	Visualizing, Inquiring, Intending, Focusing
	Energetic	Sensing, Intuiting, Balancing
	Compression	Pressing/Pushing
	Expansion	Pulling
	Kinetic	Mobilizing, Letting Go, Holding/Supporting
	Gliding	Sliding/Planing

Deep Tissue Sculpting

Carol Osborne-Sheets

Sculpting is a form of deep tissue *massage* characterized by firm, constant compressions and strokes applied parallel to the muscle fibers. *Techniques* are intended to affect the deeper structures of the musculoskeletal system, the skin and more superficial *fascia* and muscles. In order to reach these deeper layers, the sculptor uses the fingertips, knuckles, elbows, forearms, heels of the hand or any bony body part as tools. Pressure is gradually applied to a tight area until a resistance is met. Constant pressure is maintained while the tissue relaxes until release is complete, or until the practitioner accepts that no further change is forthcoming. Work proceeds slowly to allow the client time to assimilate deeper pressures and the intensity of possible psychological, physical and emotional sensations.

Deep Tissue Sculpting, a sensitive, yet penetrating method of somatic therapy, is partially technical in nature. The methodology developed from experience, supported by observation, description, experimental investigations and theoretical explanations. Intuition, emotion, and empathetic connection contribute a vibrant artistry and holistic dimension.

The practitioner actually becomes a sculpting artist and carves away that which is not the essence of the human body. S/he holds a mental picture of the muscle or fascial sheath as it appears in anatomy books. Using imagination s/he intends to create myofascia that is free of bunching, constriction or disorganization. There is a sense of sinking, melting or soaking into the client's body as gradual levels of pressure and intensity warm the tissues. Any pain experienced by the client feels cleansing and doesn't produce tension or resistance. As muscle tension and fascial disorganization melt, the practitioner envisions the skeleton, thereby bringing consciousness to the bone. Muscles, *fascia* and joints lengthen as the body elongates. Imagining such changes encourages the body to respond.

Deep Tissue Sculpting

TouchAbilities®

Technique	Component	Skill
Compression	Breathing	Tracking, Directing
	Cognitive	Visualizing, Intending, Focusing, Transmitting, Inquiring
	Energetic	Sensing, Intuiting, Balancing
	Compression	Pressing
Compression-to-Follow	Breathing	Tracking, Directing
	Cognitive	Visualizing, Intending, Focusing, Transmitting, Inquiring
	Energetic	Sensing, Intuiting, Balancing
	Compression	Pressing/Pushing
	Gliding	Planing

Feldenkrais Method®

Jill Goldman

The Feldenkrais Method® is an experiential process that exploits the infinite human potential for learning and change. Through exercise sequences, called Awareness Through Movement® lessons, and the hands-on *component*, called Functional Integration® lessons, people are able to recognize and unlearn dysfunctional movement patterns, and learn new ways to move easily, efficiently and comfortably. Moshe Feldenkrais set the goal to "Make the impossible possible, the possible easy, and the easy elegant." Clients are referred to as pupils or students.

Awareness Through Movement® (ATM) consists of verbally directed, gentle exercise lessons, approximately 45 minutes in length, involving sophisticated movement sequences. The lessons are designed to heighten awareness and to access the sensorimotor processes of the brain, including attention, perception, imagination and cognition. During the lesson, participants are encouraged to reduce muscular effort. ATM lessons are designed to teach people how they organize themselves to perform basic functions, such as sitting, standing, walking, turning and moving through the full spectrum of daily activities. One goal of the lessons is for people to learn easier, more efficient ways of organizing and moving. During ATM lessons the practitioner primarily employs Breathing, Cognitive, Kinetic and Energetic *techniques* to verbally guide pupils in active movement.

Functional Integration® (FI) is the hands-on, one-on-one *component* of the Feldenkrais Method®. FI lessons are performed with pupils comfortably clothed. Through subtle manipulations and passive mobilizations the practitioner facilitates change and improvements in the person. With her hands, the practitioner communicates the experience of easier, more pleasurable and functional movement. FI lessons are custom-tailored in the moment to the pupil's needs and abilities. The emphasis of the lesson is to inform, rather than to correct. This type of *BodyWork* creates the potential for permanent change due to the innate ability of people to learn and adopt new ways of usage. FI lessons are sequenced in such a way that they duplicate the directed movements of ATM utilizing *techniques* of the Kinetic Component on a passive client.

Together, the two Feldenkrais® *techniques*, ATM and FI, could possibly utilize all of the TouchAbilities® skills. The overarching intention of the Feldenkrais Method® is to help the pupil/client discover the space between stimulus and response, and between thought and action that allows for choice, change and growth in all the dimensions of human experience.

Feldenkrais Method™   TouchAbilities®

Technique	Component	Skill
Awareness Through Movement	Breathing	Directing, Tracking
	Cognitive	Focusing, Intending, Inquiring, Visualizing, Transmitting
	Energetic	Intuiting, Sensing, Balancing
	Kinetic	Mobilizing
Functional Integration	Breathing	Directing, Tracking
	Cognitive	Focusing, Intending, Inquiring, Visualizing, Transmitting
	Energetic	Intuiting, Sensing, Balancing
	Compression	Pressing/Pushing, Squeezing/Pinching
	Expansion	Lifting, Pulling, Rolling
	Kinetics	Holding/Supporting, Dropping/Letting Go, Mobilizing

Geriatric Massage

Sharon Puszko

Geriatric Massage is a form of *BodyWork* designed especially to meet the specific needs of the elderly population. Elderly refers to everyone over 65 and geriatric refers to health conditions that are commonly due to physiological wear and tear resulting from chronological aging. It is a *modality* that manipulates the soft tissues of the body to improve blood and lymph circulation, relieve pain, improve range of motion and restore *mobility*. It is also used to relieve anxiety, loneliness and depression and provide comfort to touch-deprived elderly people.

Geriatric Massage identifies three client *assessment* categories: robust, age-appropriate or frail, and uses basic *BodyWork techniques* tailored to specific health conditions and needs. There are some special considerations in designing a treatment protocol. The touch may be gentler to accommodate the more fragile client. Occasional use of stronger movements such as friction and pressure *techniques* are sometimes used to improve flexibility. Shorter sessions, which usually last no longer than 30 minutes, respect the stress on the body that a longer session might impose. The therapist must also take into consideration the impact of medications being used.

The elderly often experience a variety of age-related diseases such as Parkinson's, arthritis, diabetes or heart disease. They involve poor circulation and limited physical capability. Geriatric Massage can help maintain and improve overall health, as well as restore certain physical functions that are reduced or lost due to aging.

Addressing the client's emotional needs, Geriatric Massage is calming and pleasurable and creates a sense of acceptance and reassurance. It increases blood circulation, softens hardened muscle sections and muscle knots, eliminates spasms, and improves muscle coordination, especially in walking. It increases the excretion of toxins from the body and improves quality of sleep. In general, it improves a client's quality of life and self-esteem.

Geriatric Massage

TouchAbilities®

Technique	Component	Skill
Fluffing (consisting of effleurage light wringing & simultaneous petrissage)	Cognitive Compression Gliding	Intending Squeezing Sliding
Widening of Plantar Surface (foot work)	Expansion	Pulling, Rolling
Tree Shake (lumbar)	Kinetic Energetic Oscillation	Mobilizing Sensing Vibrating, Shaking
Wing Shake (key to chest work)	Oscillation Expansion Kinetic	Vibrating, Shaking Lifting Holding/Supporting
Three Finger Petrissage	Oscillation Expansion	Vibrating, Shaking Rolling, Lifting

Hoshino Therapy®

Dashi Kocica (for Bodhi Kocica)

Hoshino Therapy® specializes in the early detection and treatment of biomechanical pain and addresses the underlying causes of aging and patterns of wear and tear in the joints and soft tissues. The method utilizes a 270 acu-point system and ROM movements to *localize* areas of biomechanical stress, joint disequilibrium and to assess overall coordination. Through stimulation of selected acu-points using Hoshino's unique manual *techniques*, normal movement patterns and soft tissue vitality is gradually restored, relieving pain and its underlying cause. A program of daily exercise, appropriate for a client's condition, complements the therapy and is essential for complete rehabilitation and prevention of future problems.

Hoshino embodies for the therapist the goal of developing tactile sensitivity of the hands as well as the ability to detect subtle changes in soft tissue vitality, thereby identify stages of aging. Hand strength needs to be developed to apply Hoshino's unique manual *technique* of digital thumb pressure with full hand contact. This provides for efficient transmission of heat and pressure, and also protects the therapist from overuse syndromes. Proper dosage or "digital precision" is emphasized. This involves sensing and delivering the exact amount of pressure needed to revitalize the tissues, creating only a minimum of pain for the client. Mobilizing and stabilizing a joint, while stimulating points, helps to create a correct line of pull. Passive movements are used to assess ROM and joint function, and promote neuromuscular re-education and mobilization.

Hoshino Therapy® is beyond any single BodyView. From a structural perspective, it focuses on *body mechanics*— posture, joint equilibrium, tracking and line of pull. Functionally it regards the body as an integrity, with the goal of restoring harmonious coordination and minimum wear and tear to the moving parts. And energetically it works to normalize energetic flow and movement patterns through the stimulation of Hoshino's selected acupuncture points located along lines of pull.

Hoshino Therapy®   # TouchAbilities®

Technique	Component	Skill
Digital Pressure with Full Hand Contact	Compression	Pressing, Squeezing, Twisting
	Expansion	Pulling, Lifting, Rolling
	Kinetic	Holding, Mobilizing, Letting Go, Stabilizing
	Gliding	Planing, Rubbing
	Cognitive	Visualizing, Inquiring, Intending, Focusing
	Energetic	Sensing, Intuiting
Dosage/ Digital Precision	All of the above	
Cranial Suture Mobilization	All of the above plus: Oscillation	Vibration
Rhythm	Breathing	Tracking, Synchronizing
Traction	Kinetic	Holding, Mobilizing, Letting Go, Stabilizing
	Expansion	Pulling, Lifting, Rolling
Passive ROM Movement	Kinetic	Holding, Mobilizing, Letting Go, Stabilizing
	Compression	Pressing, Squeezing
	Expansion	Pulling, Lifting
	Cognitive	Visualizing, Inquiring, Intending, Focusing
	Energetic	Sensing, Intuiting
Hoshino Exercises	Kinetic	Holding, Mobilizing, Letting Go, Stabilizing
	Energetic	Sensing, Intuiting, Balancing
	Breathing	Tracking, Pacing

Hydrotherapy

Iris Burman and Sandy Friedland with chart by Steve Capellini

Hydrotherapy encompasses the use of water in any of its three forms— solid, liquid or vapor— for cleansing or therapeutic purposes. It can be taken internally and/or applied externally as a *local* or *general* full *body* treatment. Hydro *techniques* can be used to affect every aspect of the *body's* physical, emotional, mental and spiritual *domains*.

Water is vital to life. It is the key ingredient to all living functions. It contains usable minerals and is a source of energy and hydration. It serves as a transport system for nutrients, electrical impulses, energetic frequencies and chemical messages throughout the *body*. Humans, being 75% water, derive significant benefits from hydrotherapy treatments.

Water can be used in static or kinetic ways – in place or moving. Ice can be statically placed or kinetically moved back and forth over a *body* area. Liquid water can be statically applied in a compress or filled in a tub for soaking. Water becomes kinetic via jets, showers or hoses. Vapors are by their very nature kinetic.

Because water is a great conductor of temperature, a thorough understanding of the effects of hot, cold and neutral on each *body* system is key to effectively employing hydrotherapy. As stated in The Healing Energies of Water by Charlie Ryrie, "Cold is stimulating, making surface blood vessels constrict, inhibiting the biochemical reactions that cause *inflammation*. Cold water also sends blood towards the internal organs, helping them to function better. Hot water is relaxing. It dilates blood vessels, reduces blood pressure and increases blood flow to the skin and muscles, easing stiffness. It improves circulation, boosts the immune system, helps remove waste products from the *body* and sends more oxygen and nutrients into the tissues to repair damage. Alternating hot and cold water stimulates the hormonal system, reduces circulatory congestion, relieves *inflammation* and balances blood pressure. It also increases the *body's* electrical potential and therefore its ability to receive vibrations or energy."

Hydrotherapy can be used as a stand-alone treatment or in conjunction with other forms of healing or pampering. Water is an abundant natural element and water treatments are readily available at spas, health clubs, doctors' offices, *BodyWork* therapy centers, the seashore, mountain hot springs or at home.

Hydro treatments in destination and day spas are mostly geared to pampering, indulgence and relaxation. Some contemporary hydrotherapy centers feature multisensory "dream chambers" complete with underwater music and mind-expanding light shows as well as sensory deprivation flotation tanks which represent the other end of the spectrum. These centers also offer stainless steel sitz baths, needle showers, whirlpools, Jacuzzis, steam baths, saunas, cold pools, mud wraps and thalassotherapy treatments. In addition, there are many medical spas throughout the world that have historically provided "the cure" for people dealing with *chronic* debilitating illnesses. Recent developments are highlighted by the profusion of small local day spas and an expansion of the luxury hotel spa. Another current trend is toward the growth of more healing-type medically oriented facilities.

Hydrotherapy

TouchAbilities®

Technique	Component	Skill
Exfoliation	Compression	Pressing/Pushing
	Kinetic	Holding/Supporting
	Gliding	Sliding, Rubbing
Showers/Sprays/Water Pressure Massage	Compression	Pressing/Pushing
	Oscillation	Vibrating, Striking
Pools, springs, rivers, lakes, oceans, etc. (Aquatic BodyWork, water exercises, etc.)	Cognitive	Intending, Focusing, Transmitting
	Expansion	Pulling, Lifting
	Kinetic	Holding/Supporting, Mobilizing, Letting Go, Stabilizing
	Oscillation	Vibrating, Striking
	Breathing	Tracking, Directing
	Energetic	Sensing, Balancing
Baths/Soaks	Cognitive	Visualizing, Intending
	Kinetic	Holding/Supporting
	Energetic	Sensing, Balancing
Flotation Tank	Cognitive	Visualizing, Focusing, Inquiring
	Expansion	Lifting
	Kinetic	Holding/Supporting
	Energetic	Sensing, Intuiting, Balancing
	Breathing	Tracking, Directing
Heat/Cold	Cognitive	Focusing, Intending
	Energetic	Sensing, Intuiting, Balancing
	Expansion	Lifting (effects of heat)
	Compression	Pressing/Pushing (effects of cold)
Ocean Therapy/Dolphin Therapy	Cognitive	Visualizing, Focusing, Inquiring
	Energetic	Sensing, Intuiting, Balancing

Hydrotherapy (continued)

TouchAbilities®

Technique	Component	Skill
Water/Wave Vibration	Kinetic	Holding/Supporting, Mobilizing, Letting Go, Stabilizing
	Oscillation	Vibrating, Shaking
	Breathing	Tracking, Directing
Ingestion ("Taking the Waters")	Energetic	Sensing, Intuiting, Balancing
	Cognitive	Visualizing, Intending

Inside-Out Paradigm

Dale Alexander

The Inside-Out Paradigm is an approach that assists the body to reveal and resolve what is going on within the complex interactions of human physiology. The goal of the work is to kick-start the healing process by assisting the body to redistribute strain and reallocate resources.

Stress and trauma trigger the stereotypic response of contraction by the sacs, tubes and suspensory ligaments of the organ systems. This contraction, if sustained, builds tension and charge from the inside out. The building and accumulation of this internal tension requires the body to distribute the strain as widely as possible. There is a predictable sequence of the distribution whereby the strain is spread to the intrinsic muscles, then to the osseous structures and finally to the extrinsic musculature.

Acute and semi-*acute* episodes of musculoskeletal dysfunction and pain may actually serve to discharge this build-up of inner tensions. However, when clients present with *chronic* symptoms it infers that their capacity for discharge has become "stuck" or "congested" in some way.

The Inside-Out method uses a simple kinesthetic screening procedure to identify where the body is most congested or stuck. The practitioner relies on basic principles of anatomy and physiology and an attitude of "following the body" to assist the process of unraveling the matrix of energetic, neurocirculatory, visceral and biomechanical relationships.

Ironically, success is achieved when the symptom profile of the client shifts from one place to another, breaking a *chronic* pattern and eventually full function is restored and/or, when internal symptoms clarify to the point where referral to a physician is indicated. Many *chronic* musculoskeletal ailments are the body's alarm bell that stress related ailments have actually passed a tipping point, which signifies the beginning of pathology. This approach seems to clarify the body's ability to communicate this distinction.

The Inside-Out Paradigm emerged from 25 years' experience of working with all kinds of *chronic* dysfunctions. The touch *techniques* utilized are drawn from various disciplines of Osteopathic Manual Therapy, Soma Bodywork and Integrated Awareness®. More specifically, they include gentle visceral fascial releases, recoil *techniques*, muscle energy *techniques*, Counterstrain *techniques*, CranioSacral *techniques* and Integrated Awareness® energetic touch.

Inside-Out Paradigm

TouchAbilities®

Technique	Component	Skill
Gentle Visceral Fascial Release	Energetic	Sensing, Intuiting
	Compression	Pressing/Pushing
	Kinetic	Holding/Supporting
Recoil Technique	Breathing	Tracking, Directing, Pacing
	Energetic	Sensing, Intuiting, Balancing
	Compression	Pressing, Squeezing
	Expansion	Pulling, Lifting
Muscle Energy Technique	Kinetic	Holding/Supporting, Mobilizing, Stabilizing, Letting Go
	Breathing	Tracking, Directing, Pacing
	Cognitive	Visualizing, Inquiring, Intending, Focusing, Transmitting
	Compression	Pushing
Counterstrain	Breathing	Tracking, Directing
	Cognitive	Inquiring, Intending, Focusing, Transmitting
	Energetic	Sensing, Intuiting
	Compression	Pressing/Pushing, Twisting/Wringing
	Expansion	Pulling, Lifting, Rolling
	Kinetic	Holding/Supporting, Mobilizing, Stabilizing
Integrated Awareness® Energetic Touch	Breathing	Tracking, Directing, Pacing
	Cognitive	Visualizing, Inquiring, Intending, Focusing, Transmitting
	Energetic	Sensing, Intuiting, Balancing
	Compression	Pressing/Pushing, Squeezing/Pinching, Twisting/Wringing
	Kinetic	Holding/Supporting, Mobilizing, Stabilizing, Letting Go

Inside-Out Paradigm (continued)

TouchAbilities®

Technique	Component	Skill
CranioSacral Techniques	Breathing	Tracking, Directing, Pacing
	Cognitive	Visualizing, Inquiring, Intending, Focusing, Transmitting
	Energetic	Sensing, Intuiting, Balancing
	Compression	Pressing/Pushing, Squeezing/Pinching, Twisting/Wringing
	Kinetic	Holding/Supporting, Mobilizing, Stabilizing, Letting Go

Karmapa Reiki

Ernesto Ortiz

Reiki is a healing art and enlightenment system originally developed in the early 1900s by Mikao Usui. The Reiki form currently practiced in the Western world evolved from the teachings of Mrs. Hawayo Takata from the Usui lineage. The word "Reiki" is often translated to mean "Universal Life Energy" and represents enlightenment or the blending of our energy with the Universal Spirit of Creation. Reiki incorporates intent and "laying on of hands." Practitioners do not use their own energy; they let loving Universal Life Energy flow through them.

Basically, Reiki is comprised of five principles for living, a set of hand positions for treating self and others and the receiving of attunements (a ceremony performed by a Reiki teacher or "master") that reconnects a student with Reiki energy. It is not learned in books, but is part of an oral tradition passed on from person to person and heart to heart. Practitioners learn hand positions, distant healing, scanning, beaming, fluffing, raking and pulling energy; how to work on and off the *body*, identify bands of energy, send the symbols; and how to use this energy for others and themselves, animals, objects and more. It is essential to learn the chakra system, how it functions/dysfunctions and how to balance each individual chakra.

There are three levels in Reiki. Level I focuses on the physical body. Level II presents distance healing and addresses the mental and emotional bodies. Level III addresses the spiritual body and integrates the first two attunements to manifest 100% energy potential in the receiver. One also receives the master attunement and learns how to teach. Level III is called the Master Level; however this title should be claimed only after achieving a specific degree of wisdom and expertise.

There are various Reiki systems such as Karmapa Reiki, Shamanic Reiki, Angel Touch Reiki, Anugraha Reiki, and more. Karmapa Reiki is a healing and meditative practice using the Karmapa energy and symbols. This system is more powerful and effective because, in addition to the original Usui symbols, Karmapa Reiki teaches two more symbols in level I, an additional two symbols in level II, and one more symbol in level III. Karmapa is a Sanskrit word, that means "any action that is taken to diminish the suffering of others." It could be said that all Reiki is Karmapa because the ultimate goal is to alleviate the suffering of all sentient beings.

Karmapa Reiki   TouchAbilities®

Technique	Component	Skill
Hands on Positions	Cognitive	Visualizing, Focusing, Intending, Inquiring, Transmitting
	Energetic	Sensing, Intuiting, Balancing
	Kinetic	Holding, Supporting
Occipital Hold	Cognitive	Visualizing, Focusing, Intending, Transmitting, Inquiring
	Energetic	Sensing, Intuiting, Balancing
Hands Off Work	Cognitive	Visualizing, Focusing, Transmitting, Intending
	Energetic	Sensing, Intuiting, Balancing
Scanning	Cognitive	Focusing, Intending, Inquiring
	Energetic	Sensing, Intuiting
	Kinetic	Mobilizing
Beaming	Cognitive	Visualizing, Focusing, Transmitting, Intending
	Energetic	Balancing, Sensing
Distance Healing	Cognitive	Visualizing, Focusing, Transmitting, Intending
	Energetic	Balancing, Sensing
Chakra Balancing	Cognitive	Visualizing, Focusing, Transmitting, Intending
	Energetic	Sensing, Intuiting, Balancing
	Breathing	Tracking
	Compression	Pressing/Pushing
	Expansion	Lifting, Pulling
	Kinetic	Holding/Supporting
	Oscillation	Vibrating

LomiLomi

Paula Hamelik

"May you remember every moment of your life, the beauty, power and love you experienced at your first breath." This prayer, often spoken before a LomiLomi session, embodies both the intent and focus of Hawaii's sacred *BodyWork*. Drawing upon knowledge of psychospiritual anatomy, elemental energetics, the seven principles of healing, and the ability to balance masculine and feminine, severity and mercy, the LomiLomi practitioner endeavors to create a safe and loving environment wherein the recipient can break old patterns of holding that might span generations. With this shift, the recipient can heal old psychospiritual wounds and eventually own and celebrate that spark of The Divine that s/he truly is.

LomiLomi is characterized physically by long, flowing strokes primarily using forearms and elbows with the hands as guides. By necessity it is very oily work. Profound depth is achieved by leverage using leaning rather than pushing. This results in gentle penetration into the tissues and minimizes strain on the practitioner's body. It is also very intimate work and a primary area of focus (considered vital by most Polynesians) is the 'opu or abdomen.

LomiLomi is ideal for deep release and relaxation, as well as gaining insight into psychospiritual issues held in the body. *Contraindications* include those for Swedish Massage, however the work can be modified based on the *skill* and training of the practitioner.

The accompanying chart lists the basic manual *techniques* used in this flowing *modality*. The intentionality and energetics have not been included because, as with all ancient healing arts in which body, mind, spirit and soul have not been separated one from the other, it is understood that they permeate and drive the physical actions.

LomiLomi

TouchAbilities®

Technique	Component	Skill
Kaomi (kah-oh-mee)	Compression	Pressing
Ko (koh)	Compression	Pushing
	Expansion	Pulling
Au (ow)	Gliding	Sliding
Kahi (kah-hee)	Gliding	Planing
	Compression	Pressing
'Opa (oh-pah)	Compression	Squeezing
Ho' onaue (ho-oh-now-eh) (rocking)	Oscillation	Shaking
Ho'o'unu (ho-oh-ew-new)	Oscillation	Shaking
	Expansion	Pulling
Kuolo (koo-oh-low)	Compression	Pushing
Mahiki (mah-hee-kee)	Oscillation	Vibrating
Wekeweke (veh-keh-veh-keh)	Gliding	Rubbing
	Compression	Pushing

Medical Massage

Ralph Stephens

Medical Massage is, in reality, more of an orientation than a particular set of *techniques*. Its focus is to work with clients who have medical or rehabilitative considerations. This approach is a synthesis of education, training, experience, dedication, humility and intuition. It is an integrative treatment, which can include *massage* therapy, stretching and joint mobilization to create a unique protocol for each client. Many existing *modalities* of soft tissue manipulation and body/mind support effectively address its goals.

Medical Massage IS NOT *general* relaxation *massage*; it is manual therapy applied to a specific body area and focused on the primary pathology of a client's chief complaint. While it can be given as a full body treatment, it is most commonly delivered to an anatomic region, based on joint and soft tissue findings after taking a complete case history, a thorough posture analysis and performing palpatory *assessments* of the tissues. Other *assessment techniques* may also be used including range of motion tests, orthopedic muscle testing and gait analysis.

Medical Massage may or may not be performed under a physician's prescription or referral. A physician's diagnosis of the condition being treated is desirable but not required. While Medical Massage may be performed in a hospital, medical clinic, or interdisciplinary practice, it may also take place in a private office, a *BodyWork* therapy clinic, or even on-site at a client's location.

Medical Massage is an advanced discipline of *BodyWork* therapy. What distinguishes Medical Massage therapists is additional knowledge of *techniques*, injuries, pathologies, medical terminology, equipment and procedures. This expanded knowledge is generally taught in post entry-level continuing education programs. However, some entry-level schools now offer Medical Massage as advanced level electives while others make it the focus of their entire curriculum.

Although Medical Massage therapists may utilize almost any *BodyWork modality*, the more commonly used methods include connective tissue *massage*, neuromuscular therapy, stretching and joint mobilization *techniques*, periosteal *massage* and segment-reflex *massage*. There are specific Medical Massage courses that teach the expanded knowledge base of Medical Massage. The classic *techniques* utilized in Medical Massage are referred to by the classic Western European terminology recognized in medical texts and dictionaries.

Medical Massage works in conjunction with the medical *techniques* and protocols of other systems of manual therapy, including medical acupuncture, chiropractic, exercise, etc., and can be integrated into orthopedic and physical therapy protocols.

Medical Massage

TouchAbilities®

Technique	Component	Skill
Compression	Compression	Pressing
Deep Friction	Compression	Pushing
	Gliding	Rubbing
Effleurage	Compression	Pushing
	Gliding	Sliding, Planing
Nerve Strokes	Gliding	Sliding
Petrissage	Compression	Squeezing/Pinching, Twisting/Wringing
Stretching (muscle, tendon, fascia)	Kinetic	Mobilizing, Holding
	Compression	Pushing
	Expansion	Pulling, Rolling
	Gliding	Planing
Traction	Expansion	Pulling
Range of Motion (joint mobilization)	Expansion	Pulling, Lifting
	Kinetic	Mobilizing
Superficial Friction	Compression	Pushing, Wringing
	Gliding	Rubbing
Sustained Pressure	Compression	Pushing, Pinching
	Kinetic	Holding
Tapotement	Oscillation	Striking
Vibration	Oscillation	Shaking, Vibrating

NOTE: Medical Massage therapists often incorporate the Cognitive Component *skills* of Inquiring, Intending, Visualizing, Focusing and Transmitting, the Breathing Component *skills* of Tracking, Directing and Pacing as well as the Energetic Component *skills* of Sensing, Intuiting, and Balancing. *SenseAbilities*™ are also employed as Medical Massage therapists usually work with some form of S.O.A.P. notes and must communicate with both the client and other health care providers.

MotherMassage®

Elaine Stillerman

MotherMassage®, a combination of *BodyWork techniques* developed by Elaine Stillerman, is designed to safely and comfortably treat women during pregnancy, labor and postpartum recovery. Historically, this type of *BodyWork* has been integrated into social systems of most tribal societies. Supported by scientific understanding of the process, MotherMassage® brings this important work into the modern world.

Seeking to realign the body to provide maximum structural integrity and function, this system works with the dynamic structural compensations and the shifting center of gravity experienced during pregnancy. Particular attention is paid to strengthening and maintaining the core abdominal muscles that play a major role in lumbar stability and postural support. MotherMassage® also addresses the dramatic metabolic, *systemic* and emotional changes of pregnancy and focuses on safely reducing the discomforts associated with them.

MotherMassage® labor support is attuned to a woman's ever-changing physical and emotional needs as labor progresses. It can be provided by a professional assisting at the birth or by the birth partner. The treatment focuses on offering comfort measures to minimize labor pain, treat back labor, provide important emotional support and speed up the labor process. *Massage* between contractions consists of long, gliding strokes to reduce the waste products within the muscles and to reoxygenate the blood. During contractions, more *localized techniques* are used, such as counterpressure, pelvic squeeze, sacral lift or pressing specific acupuncture points to hasten labor.

Postpartum *massage* addresses the new mother's needs at three different time periods during the recovery process. Treatment within the first few hours and days after the birth mainly enhances elimination and cleansing processes that naturally occur early in postpartum. During the traditional 6-week puerperium period, muscle-balancing *techniques* are introduced while treatment continues to minimize fatigue and address nursing issues. As a new mother moves further away from the birth, the long-term physiological and emotional effects of pregnancy and labor are treated to prevent *chronic* discomfort and related or referred stress patterns.

MotherMassage®   ## TouchAbilities®

Technique	Component	Skill
Observation	Cognitive	Intending, Focusing
Sensing	Energetic	Sensing, Intuiting, Balancing
	Cognitive	Visualizing, Inquiring, Intending, Focusing, Transmitting
Muscle Elongation & Soft Tissue Release & Joint Decompression & Structural Alignment	Gliding	Sliding, Rubbing
	Expansion	Pulling, Lifting
	Compression	Pressing/Pushing, Squeezing
	Kinetic	Holding/Supporting, Mobilizing, Stabilizing, Letting Go/Dropping
Lymphatic Drainage	Compression	(Light) Pressing/Pushing, Squeezing
	Gliding	(Light) Sliding, Rubbing
Joint Mobilization	Kinetic	Holding/Supporting, Mobilizing
	Compression	Pressing
	Expansion	Pulling
Muscle & Joint Traction	Kinetic	Holding, Supporting, Stabilizing, Mobilizing
	Cognitive	Focusing, Transmitting
Trigger Point Release	Compression	Pressing/Pushing
	Kinetic	Holding
Proprioceptive Techniques	Compression	Pressing/Pushing
	Kinetic	Holding
Postural/Gravitational Release	Kinetic	Supporting, Stabilizing, Letting Go/Dropping
	Compression	Pressing/Pushing
Scar Massage	Compression	Twisting/Wringing
	Expansion	Pulling, Lifting, Rolling
	Gliding	Planing, Rubbing
	Kinetic	Mobilizing

MotherMassage® (continued)

TouchAbilities®

Technique	Component	Skill
Energy Work	Energetic	Sensing, Intuiting, Balancing
	Cognitive	Visualizing, Intending, Focusing, Transmitting
Pelvic Squeeze, Medial Compression	Kinetic	Holding/ Supporting, Letting Go
Pelvic Tilt	Kinetic	Holding/ Supporting, Letting Go
Sacral Lift	Kinetic	Holding/ Supporting, Letting Go
Holding	Kinetic	Holding/ Supporting
Rocking	Oscillation	(Gentle) Shaking
Attuned Breathing	Breathing	Pacing, Directing

Multi-Dimensional Movement Arts®

Sandy Friedland

Imagine yourself in the womb. It's warm and nurturing. You feel totally safe and supported. You feel your breath, your heartbeat. You hear your inner voice. Gentle *waves* caress your *body*. You are one with the flows and *rhythms* of movement. You're in a *state* of dynamic balance. You are pure potentiality. This is ecstasy!

Multi-Dimensional Movement Arts®, water version, is the art of using movement in the medium of water to create dynamic balance. Specific actions, patterns and *waveforms* promote reorganization, re-education, rehabilitation, relaxation and rejuvenation. This continuous process of attunement leads to heightened *states* of awareness and bliss.

In a typical MDMA® session, the client is supported by strategically placed flotation devices and moved through water that is at body temperature. Trained practitioner/s treat a person by playing with various interconnections and influences of circles, spirals and infinity signs. Not only do these actions promote vitality and optimal health, they also induce deep relaxation, release endorphins, heighten awareness, alter consciousness and produce euphoria. It is exponentially powerful and exquisite when the client receives a two-on-one session as two therapists team up to deliver the movements.

A *body* in water is buoyant. The liquid environment changes auditory experience. One can move freely without consciously engaging muscles. Sensations of time, space and distance are distorted and experience is shifted from ordinary reality. This affects a person on many different levels: memories are jogged, holding patterns released, *body* parts awakened and awareness stimulated. The work supports and encourages gentle surrender. The ultimate goal of MDMA® is freedom of movement on all levels– physical, emotional, mental and spiritual– so that one resonates with his/her optimal frequency.

Buoyancy and hydrostatic qualities bring a different dynamic to the practitioner's movements of lunging, twisting, leaning, moving back and forth, up and down and from side to side. Developing good *body mechanics* is key to the transfer of energy from practitioner to client as they both move through the water. MDMA® is especially easy on the therapist and each session also supports his/her own balance and well-being. An added bonus of MDMA® is that people can use the flotation devices and generate their own movements and actions to administer a self-treatment.

MDMA®

TouchAbilities®

Technique	Component	Skill
Wave Making (circles, spirals & infinity signs)	Breathing	Tracking, Directing, Pacing
	Cognitive	Visualizing, Inquiring, Intending
Navigating	Cognitive	Focusing, Transmitting
	Energetic	Sensing, Intuiting, Balancing
	Compression	Pressing/Pushing, Squeezing/Pinching, Twisting
	Expansion	Pulling, Lifting, Rolling
	Kinetic	Holding/Supporting, Mobilizing, Stabilizing
	Oscillation	Vibrating, Shaking
Throwing	Kinetics	Mobilizing
	Compression	Pushing
Whirling/Swinging	Expansion	Pulling
Cradling	Kinetic	Holding/Supporting, Stabilizing
	Breathing	Tracking, Directing, Pacing
	Energetic	Sensing, Intuiting, Balancing
	Cognitive	Visualizing, Inquiring, Intending, Focusing, Transmitting
Scraping	Compression	Pressing/Pushing
	Gliding	Planing
	Kinetics	Stabilizing
Ironing	Gliding	Sliding, Planing
	Compression	Pushing
	Expansion	Pulling
Curling	Compression	Squeezing/Pinching, Twisting/Wringing
	Expansion	Pulling, Rolling

MDMA® (continued)   TouchAbilities®

Technique	Component	Skill
Docking	Kinetic	Mobilizing
Rebounding	Expansion	Pulling
	Compression	Pushing

The above MDMA® *techniques* denote a starting point for creating *waves* and movement patterns. They represent core actions available for working on clients in the water. This is not a comprehensive list because an MDMA® session is a constant, ever-changing, ongoing, in-the-moment, exploratory cocreation.

Myofascial Therapy

Pete Whitridge

Myofascial Therapy is also known as Myofascial Release, Connective Tissue Massage and Bindegewebsmassage. The foundational principle of myofascial *BodyWork* is to melt and soften the fascia surrounding the tissue being treated. According to Dean Juhan and others, *fascia* (connective tissue) responds to pressure and heat by melting and becoming more liquid. This quality and ability to change from gel (solid) to sol (liquid) is known as *thixotropy*. Experienced therapists report feeling the tissues softening or melting under their hands when the *fascia* changes. The client often reports more freedom of movement and fluidity in the surrounding tissues.

Another property of *fascia* is its ability to act as a liquid crystal. Researchers have found that *fascia* emits a small electrical charge when pressure or heat is applied to it. This electrical charge, known as piezoelectricity, stimulates the adjacent tissues and causes them to soften and change (*thixotropy*). This system is in intimate relationship with the muscles, ligaments and tendons. Changes in muscle tone, pressure on a joint capsule, or pulling a limb can cause the connective tissues to change from gel to sol and vice versa.

Myofascial therapy practitioners tend to work obliquely to the tissues (30–45 degrees), pulling and lengthening the *fascia* in relationship to its underlying muscle. Individual muscles are treated by lengthening, spreading and defining the *fascia* around them. The melting of *fascia* gives individual muscles more space and fluidity in relation to the surrounding tissues. It is vital for therapists to know the direction of pull of the muscle fibers and the action of those fibers on the bones and joints connected to them. Moving and melting the *fascia* in opposition to habitual patterns can help create more optimal patterns. Also, new neurological inputs can be integrated through the brain back into the muscles, ligaments and tendons. Myofascial *techniques* can be incorporated in any treatment session and are the foundational applications utilized in structural integrative *modalities* such as Rolfing, Structural Integration, Soma or Core Bodywork.

Myofascial Therapy

TouchAbilities®

Technique	Component	Skill
Assessment of Restrictions	Compression Expansion	Pushing Pulling
Effleurage— surface stroke for lengthening, broadening & definition	Gliding	Sliding
Effleurage— deeper stroke to effect deeper tissues for lengthening, broadening & definition	Gliding	Planing
Joint Mobilization	Kinetics	Holding/Supporting, Mobilizing, Stabilizing

Neuromuscular Therapy American™ Version

Judith Delany

Neuromuscular therapy (NMT) addresses the person as a whole, by broadly considering biochemical, biomechanical and psychosocial influences on a client's *state* of health. While most NMT practitioners will use manual methods to influence primarily biomechanical factors, treatment through any one or combination of these categories can usually make some change in a person's wellness *state*. Synergistic combinations can be profound.

Neuromuscular Therapy American™ version has a broad impact on the body. It specifically focuses to reduce ischemia within myofascial tissue as well as deactivate trigger points (TrPs) and, where possible, uncover the cause of their formation. It will consider and relieve nerve entrapment and/or compression possibilities and assess and influence postural alignment. Additionally, it aims to enhance well-being through nutritional awareness and reduce the effects of emotional stress.

Neuromuscular Therapy commonly uses applications of effleurage, friction, digital compression, myofascial release (MFR) through manual light traction of specific tissues, muscle energy *techniques* such as passive and active stretching, Positional Release and a variety of hydrotherapies. Additionally, an effort is made by both practitioner and client to discover the causes of primary and secondary dysfunctions. Where possible, causes are removed or altered (new chair, orthoses, awareness of head position, daily active stretching, relaxation methods, etc.) and new habits of use suggested.

When forces, such as shearing, heat, or vibration, are introduced to fascial tissue, its ground substance displays a unique property, called *thixotropy*, that allows it to change its *state* from a solid to a more liquid form. If left immobile and undisturbed it returns to a more solid *state* over a period of time, and movement eventually ceases due to solidification of synovium and connective tissue. A wide range of therapeutic interventions can be applied by the practitioner and/or the patient in an attempt to temporarily change the *state* of the ground substance from gelatinous-like (which limits movement) to a more watery, flexible solute *state*. These may include the introduction of energy through muscular activity (active or passive movement provided by activity or stretching); soft tissue manipulation (provided by specific *BodyWork techniques*); heat (hydrotherapies, manual friction); vibration (manually or mechanically applied); and nutritional changes (including fluid intake).

Neuromuscular Therapy requires thought and intuition on the part of the practitioner as to which applications to use, in what order to apply them, and how much is enough yet not too much for the client's system to effectively handle. The practitioner's role may be to alleviate the stress burden as far as possible, to lighten the load, or to work toward more efficient handling of the adaptive load. It also includes teaching and encouraging the individual to alter daily habits.

Neuromuscular Therapy American™ Version

TouchAbilities®

Technique	Component	Skill
Effleurage	Gliding	Sliding
Friction	Gliding	Rubbing (subsurface), Planing
Vibration	Oscillation	Vibrating
Digital Compression	Compression	Pressing/Pushing
Tissue Compression	Compression	Squeezing/Pinching, Twisting/Wringing
Tissue Mobilization	Expansion Compression	Pulling, Lifting, Rolling Twisting/Wringing, Pressing/Pushing
Light Traction	Kinetics Expansion	Mobilizing Pulling, Lifting
Passive/Active Stretching	Kinetics	Mobilizing, Stabilizing
Positional Release	Kinetics	Holding/Supporting
Structure Balance	Kinetics	Stabilizing
Tapotement	Oscillation	Striking, Shaking
Respiratory Rehabilitation	Breathing	Tracking, Directing
Client Assessment	Cognitive Energetic	Visualizing, Inquiring, Focusing Sensing, Intuiting, Balancing
Client Education	Cognitive	Transmitting, Intending, Focusing, Inquiring

Neuromuscular Therapy

Pete Whitridge

The philosophy and intention of Neuromuscular Therapy is to help reduce pain in injured tissues and help reset and recalibrate muscle tonus through contact with trigger points. The essential ingredient in working with this *modality* is the *palpation* of trigger points (Tps) within the muscle tissue. The NMT therapist uses pressure and gliding to identify Tps within the soft tissues. This pressure is usually applied downward in a perpendicular (90 degree) direction and will vary from location to location as dictated by the needs of the client. It may cause a sensory input that is interpreted as "pain." The painful area may be ischemic and thickened due to injury or trauma. Generally, Tps tend to soften and melt when pressure is applied, which increases the resting length of the muscle fiber. Then the Golgi tendon organs reset, and *fascia* softens to accommodate the newly lengthened muscle bundle. Too much pressure will cause the client to recoil and possibly reduce the effectiveness of the application; too little pressure and the client's sensory inputs to the brain may remain unchanged.

NMT works through the body/mind connection. A client may not report soreness or tenderness until the tissues are manipulated. Contact may cause feelings/sensations of tension or pain in the conscious realm. This neural firing at the contact point causes stimulation up the neural chain until the brain receives the message and sends out a motor neuron message to adjust to the new stimulus. After a few minutes of sustained pressure and even slow friction, the muscle, ligament, or tendon may feel completely free of Tps.

Therapists with refined touch *skills* palpate small areas of a muscle group to probe for Tps. This exploration can be assisted by verbal interaction and direction from the receiver. Including clients in the *feedback loop* is key to successful treatment. In fact, the client should be directing the treatment for optimal results. Tips such as "a little more to the right" or "less pressure, please" complete an energetic loop as the client helps the therapist "press it just right" and the therapist helps the client "feel it just right." Using controlled breathing *techniques* can also help the client "connect" with the area being treated.

There is often discussion about referral patterns and referred pain sensations. Referred pain does not have to be present to treat a Tp, however, dermatomes and enervation patterns are helpful in locating sources of pain especially in cases of nerve entrapment or compression. Referral patterns can help the therapist determine from which nerve level a problem arises and assist clients in understanding their pain, especially if that pain is distant from the spot being treated.

Neuromuscular Therapy

TouchAbilities®

Technique	Component	Skill
Effleurage	Gliding	Sliding, Planing
Petrissage	Compression	Pushing/Pressing, Squeezing/Pinching, Twisting/Wringing
	Expansion	Lifting, Pulling, Rolling
Compression of Tps (thumb/fingers-compression)	Compression	Pushing/Pressing
Open Fist— Static Pressure	Compression	Pushing/Pressing
Elbow— Slow Friction	Gliding	Rubbing
Friction of Lesion in Tendon or Ligament	Compression	Pressing
	Gliding	Rubbing
Joint Mobilization	Kinetics	Holding/Supporting, Mobilizing, Stabilizing

Orthopedic Massage

James Waslaski

Orthopedic Massage involves therapeutic *assessment*, manipulation, and movement of the locomotor soft tissues to reduce or eliminate pain and dysfunction. A unique multidisciplinary approach is utilized to restore structural balance throughout the body. The focus is prevention and rehabilitation of musculoskeletal dysfunctions, *chronic* pain and sports injuries. Primary applications include functional *assessment*, myofascial release, Positional Release, Neuromuscular Therapy, scar tissue mobilization *techniques*, neuromuscular re-education, myoskeletal alignment, joint capsule work, PNF stretching, strengthening, and specific client home care protocols. The goal is to lengthen shortened muscle groups around each joint, strengthen weak opposing muscle groups and increase joint space throughout the entire body. This eliminates myofascial pain patterns, and neuromuscular patterns or trigger points. Practitioners integrate as many advanced *BodyWork* disciplines as possible and stay extremely focused on the client as a whole. Emotional guarding and changes in breathing patterns are respected and all protocols are implemented pain free.

Orthopedic Massage, an advanced discipline in the rapidly growing field of Medical Massage, is performed with the intent to improve medical conditions or pathologies that have been diagnosed by a physician. Many special *assessment* tests commonly performed by other health care practitioners such as physical therapists are included in Orthopedic Massage training. Orthopedic Massage practitioners address *chronic* pain and other injury conditions with emphasis on understanding and correcting the cause and pathology of each specific condition. The session begins with detailed history taking and an ongoing process of evaluation, which allows the practitioner to match the appropriate application to the exact underlying condition. Focus is on structural balance of the entire body and the treatment plan is based on information obtained in the initial *assessment*. Medical precautions are respected, based on information gathered in the special tests and initial history. Most importantly, clients are given an individually designed home care program, based on the *assessment* and treatment of their specific condition. Clients are also taught to change or eliminate patterns that cause their pain. This may involve changing the *ergonomics* of a work station, shifting postural patterns, eliminating repetitive motion patterns when possible, daily stretching focused on *chronically* shortened muscle groups, proper nutrition, minimizing stress, etc.

Participants in Orthopedic Massage seminars include *massage* therapists, athletic trainers, physical therapists, occupational therapists, chiropractors, osteopaths, physicians, nurses, personal trainers and others.

Orthopedic Massage

TouchAbilities®

Technique	Component	Skill
Client Assessment	Cognitive	Visualizing, Inquiring, Focusing
	Energetic	Sensing, Intuiting, Balancing
Evaluation/ROM	Energetic	Sensing, Balancing
	Kinetics	Mobilizing, Stabilizing
	Cognitive	Visualizing, Inquiring
Special Tests	Kinetics	Holding/Supporting, Stabilizing, Mobilizing
	Compression	Pressing/Pushing
	Expansion	Pulling, Lifting, Rolling
Effleurage	Gliding	Sliding
	Energetic	Sensing
	Cognitive	Inquiring
Myofascial Release	Compression	Pushing
	Expansion	Pulling
	Kinetic	Mobilizing
Tissue Compression	Compression	Pressing/Pushing
Digital Compression	Compression	Pressing/Pushing
Cross-Fiber Friction	Gliding	Planing, Rubbing
	Compression	Pushing
Positional Release	Kinetic	Holding/Supporting
Respiratory Evaluation	Breathing	Tracking, Directing
Myoskeletal Alignment	Kinetics	Holding/Supporting, Mobilizing, Stabilizing
Structural Balance	Kinetics	Mobilizing, Stabilizing

Orthopedic Massage (continued)

TouchAbilities®

Technique	Component	Skill
Active/ PNF Stretching	Kinetics	Mobilizing, Stabilizing
	Compression	Pressing/Pushing
	Expansion	Pulling
Strengthening	Kinetics	Supporting, Mobilizing
	Compression	Pressing/Pushing
	Expansion	Pulling
Client Education	Cognitive	Transmitting, Intending, Focusing, Visualizing, Inquiring

PetMassage™, Ltd.

Jonathan Rudinger

PetMassage™ practitioners are trained to recognize, support and reinforce an animal's innate ability to self-heal. *Assessment techniques* include the use of pendulums, visual observation, *palpation* and muscle testing. PetMassage™ treatments cover physical rehabilitation and wellness maintenance as well as behavioral problems, which can range from separation anxiety, aggression and shyness to grieving and depression. Each touch is a request for permission to continue and establishes trust between the animal and therapist.

Generally, various *BodyWork techniques* are used to warm the tissues. For specific treatments regarding *chronic* pathologies such as hip dysplasia and osteoarthritis, or *acute* injuries, postsurgical rehabilitation, gait patterning and behavior modification, PetMassage™ uses variations on assistive and resistive ROM, Positional Release and traditional acupressure on acupoints and along meridians. It also incorporates cross-fiber scratching, *fascia* and osteo realignment, and healing touch for chakra/energy balancing. The physical work realigns and repositions *fascia*, muscles, tendons, bones and internal organs, along with their associated habit patterns.

Touching an animal with your hands and/or with intention brings attention and awareness to all parts of its body. Light touch brings awareness to the coat and upper layers of connective tissue and surrounding superficial muscles. Stronger pressure heightens awareness of deeper muscles, tendons, joints and ligaments. Joint mobilization promotes body-movement awareness and gives the animal permission to explore movement and rediscover its "place of comfort."

All animals are hard-wired to be outwardly focused and to react in different ways for survival, so each one has individual touch requirements. To effectively support an animal's innate tendency toward *homeostasis* and potential for self-correction, PetMassage™ practitioners learn to respect the unique response of each breed and species. It is important to work with each one at its level of understanding, to interact with appropriate touch, body language, *body mechanics* and psychic communication.

The PetMassage™ Institute also features PetMassage™ WaterWork. The buoyancy factor and fluidity of water provides an animal with a different sense of awareness regarding muscular and emotional response.

There is a growing acceptance and demand for PetMassage™. It is possible that within 10 years there will be as many animal *BodyWork* practitioners as dog groomers and trainers combined!

PetMassage™, Ltd.

TouchAbilities®

Technique	Component	Skill
Visual Assessment of Gait & Behavior	Breathing	Tracking
	Energy	Sensing, Intuiting
Obtain Permission	Cognitive	Visualizing, Inquiring, Focusing, Transmitting
Body Language	Energetic	Sensing, Intuiting
Monitoring/Adjustment	Kinetics	Mobilizing
Hook Up/Presence	Energetic	Sensing, Intuiting
	Cognitive	Transmitting
Body/Mind Integration	Cognitive	Visualizing, Inquiring, Focusing, Transmitting
	Energetic	Sensing, Intuiting, Balancing
Assessment (for tissue quality & animal receptivity)	Kinetics	Holding/Supporting, Mobilizing Letting Go/Dropping
	Oscillation	Vibrating, Shaking
Warm tissues	Gliding	Rubbing
Reflex Responses (of fascia & behaviors)	Compression	Pressing/Pushing
	Breathing	Tracking, Directing
	Kinetic	Holding/Supporting, Letting Go, Mobilizing, Stabilizing
Respiratory Enhancement	Oscillation	Striking
Tapotement/Cupping/Slapping	Oscillation	Striking
	Expansion	Pulling
	Cognitive	Visualizing, Intending
Skin Rolling	Expansion	Pulling, Rolling
Joint Mobilization	Kinetics	Holding/Supporting, Mobilizing, Stabilizing Letting Go/Dropping

PetMassage™, Ltd. (continued)

TouchAbilities®

Technique	Component	Skill
Positional Release	Energetic	Sensing, Intuiting, Balancing
Unwinding	Kinetics	Holding/Supporting, Mobilizing, Stabilizing
	Expansion	Pulling, Lifting, Rolling
	Compression	Pushing, Twisting
Side-to-side Rocking	Compression	Pressing/Pushing
	Kinetics	Mobilizing, Letting Go
	Oscillation	Shaking
Lymphatic Drainage	Gliding	Sliding
	Kinetics	Mobilizing, Letting Go
	Breathing	Tracking
Caudal to Cranial, Side-to-Side & Contralateral Holding	Kinetics	Holding/Supporting
Scratching	Gliding	Sliding
Pendulum Assessment	Energetic	Sensing, Intuiting
Chakra Balancing	Energetic	Sensing, Intuiting
Energy Jumpstart (cross-fiber scratching)	Gliding	Rubbing, Planing
Connect the Dots	Gliding	Sliding
	Energetic	Sensing, Intuiting
Grounding Nerve Strokes	Gliding	Sliding
Thanking Animal	Breathing	Tracking
Farewell Blessing	Energetic	Sensing, Intuiting
	Cognitive	Transmitting

Positional Release

Patrick Fay

Positional Release is a type of soft tissue therapy that involves total body evaluation and treatment using body "positions of comfort" and tender points to resolve dysfunction and/or pain. The physiological effects of this approach are neurological and muscular. The ultimate goal is to correct imbalances in the musculoskeletal system to improve function and health.

The practitioner puts the client's body in a position where it comes to ease, and then maintains it in that position while tissue barriers release and holding patterns shift. This gives the body an opportunity to change the degree of tension held in muscles, tendons, ligaments and myofascial tissue. Influencing the settings of muscles and joints in positions of guarding or splinting gives valuable access to the nervous system. It provides for physical, emotional and mental releases that relate to barriers of resistance that the body mounts in its attempt to adapt.

Positional Release taps into the body/mind connection and makes the efficient, simple, technically uncomplicated access into this system a practical reality.

Applying Positional Release involves positions of the joint that affects a muscle in spasm or pain. A position of ease is sought and held for 60-90 seconds followed by a gentle traction of that joint. Generally, the client remains clothed.

A form of osteopathy, Positional Release originated from the work of Dr. Lawrence Jones. This gentle, non-invasive method is directed toward pain control, releases muscle spasm and changes *chronic* body postures. Safe and effective for a broad range of clients, it is time efficient and enhances all other types of *BodyWork*.

Positional Release

TouchAbilities®

Technique	Component	Skill
Sensing Position of Ease	Cognitive Energetic	Focusing, Inquiring, Transmitting Sensing
Positioning	Kinetic	Holding/Supporting, Mobilizing
Gentle Traction (lengthening)	Kinetic Expansion	Mobilizing Pulling, Lifting
Crowding	Compression	Pressing/Pushing

Reflexology

David Allan

Reflexology is a practice based on the principle that manual pressure with specific thumb and finger *techniques* applied to the hands and feet will create physiological, chemical and emotional changes throughout the body. In Reflexology, an overlay of the *body* image is positioned over both the hands and feet. Stimulation to hand and foot points reflexively affects corresponding body parts and can produce positive health benefits.

At face value we have appendages with five digits attached that are made for touching, feeling, standing and walking. Looking more closely at the hands and feet, an entire world emerges. There is a display of lines, colors, toe and finger shapes, skin texture and temperature, as well as sensations as pressure is applied. Healthy hands and feet should not be tender to firm pressure and when they are, it's a warning sign that the health of the hands and feet or the overall body is compromised.

From a holistic perspective, the body functions as a whole and is therefore affected by everything we do and say. Reflexologists not only see and evaluate the body through the body image on the hands and feet, their direct application of pressure to specific points reflexively affects the entire body.

Reflexology is versatile and simple to use as a self-help *modality*. It is a wellness and therapeutic practice that brings relief to many ailments and provides important sensory stimulation at the point of application. It is noninvasive and provides nourishing pressure and joint movements to everyday "abused hands and feet," relieving them of *local* pent-up stress and reducing overall stress levels throughout the body.

Reflexology

TouchAbilities®

Technique	Component	Skill
Thumb & Finger Walking	Cognitive	Intending, Focusing, Transmitting
	Compression	Pushing, Squeezing/Pinching
	Expansion	Rolling
	Kinetic	Holding/Supporting, Stabilizing
Thumb & Finger Pressing	Cognitive	Intending, Focusing, Transmitting
	Compression	Pushing
	Expansion	Pulling, Lifting
	Kinetic	Holding/Supporting, Stabilizing
Rotation on a Point	Cognitive	Intending, Focusing, Transmitting
	Compression	Pushing/Pressing
	Kinetic	Holding/Supporting, Stabilizing
Thumb & Finger Rolling	Cognitive	Intending, Focusing, Transmitting
	Compression	Pushing
	Expansion	Pulling, Lifting
	Kinetic	Holding/Supporting, Stabilizing

Reflexology Works™

Ed Wilson

Reflexology is a body therapy in which *palpation* and thumb and finger compression is applied to specific reflex points on the feet and hands that relate to organs, glands and systems of the body. Pressing these points promotes relaxation, reduces pain, improves circulation and lessens the impact of stress-related illnesses and emotional disorders.

Reflexology Works™ has a strong foundation in the system originally created in the 1930s by Eunice Ingham. This more recent interpretation of the traditional Ingham method has some significant, recognizable differences. Expanding on the tradition of focusing only on the feet and hands, Reflexology Works™ includes compression, kneading, friction and shaking of the legs, feet, arms and hands. A session begins with visualization, *affirmation* and specific attention to breathing. The soft tissue manipulations and larger passive movements promote the flow of energy through the ten "zones" of the body in order to stimulate self-healing and a greater sense of balance.

Warm-up and stretching movements prepare the feet and hands for more specific thumb and finger walking. These *techniques* are interspersed throughout the session and serve as a change of pace for both the client and therapist. While no tools are used during a treatment, clients are encouraged to work with a footsie roller, golf ball or other round objects, as part of their self-care maintenance.

While there are a number of theories about how reflexology works, Reflexology Works™ is based on the following precepts. Pressure applied to specific reflex points (receptors) signals the brain to respond by producing pain-suppressing chemicals to alter the pain response. Also, persistent pressure opens up energy blockages and breaks up accumulated matter enabling it to be absorbed into the blood and lymph streams to eventually be released as waste products. Additionally, the placebo effect suggests that individuals who are familiar with this form of therapy, and believe in the ability of the practitioner, experience positive reinforcement and are helped by this treatment, which further supports their belief.

During this 30-60 minute session, the client lies on a *BodyWork* table or reclines in a Reflexology chair and remains fully clothed except for bare feet, legs and arms. Generally, no lubricant is used, but cream or lotion may be applied during a more *general* foot *massage* offered as a final touch.

Reflexology Works™   TouchAbilities®

Technique	Component	Skill
Breathing	Breathing	Tracking, Directing, Pacing
Visualizing	Cognitive	Visualizing, Focusing, Intending
Affirming	Cognitive	Focusing
Warm-up & Stretch	Compression Kinetic	Pressing/Pushing, Twisting/Wringing Holding/Supporting, Mobilizing, Stabilizing
Flicking	Oscillation Kinetic	Shaking Mobilizing
Thumb & Finger Walking	Compression	Pressing/Pushing, Squeezing/Pinching
Hook In & Back Up	Compression	Pressing/Pushing
Pinpointing	Compression	Pressing/Pushing
Joint Movements	Compression Expansion Kinetic	Pressing/Pushing, Twisting/Wringing Pulling/Lifting Holding/Supporting, Mobilizing, Stabilizing
Plantar Softening	Compression Kinetic	Pressing/Pushing Holding/Supporting, Mobilizing, Stabilizing
Traction	Kinetic Expansion	Mobilizing, Stabilizing Pulling/Lifting
Fintertip Rolling	Compression Gliding	Pressing Planing, Rubbing
Tapotement	Oscillation	Striking, Shaking
Solar Plexus Point Pressure	Compression	Pressing/Pushing
Client Education/Homework	Cognitive Compression	Visualizing, Inquiring, Intending, Transmitting Pressing/Pushing

Shiatsu

Bob Lunior

Shiatsu is a Japanese *modality* derived from Chinese Medicine which incorporates the concepts of body, mind, emotion and spirit in all its actions and intentions. It is a healing *modality* focused on bringing these elements into balance and wholeness. In a *state* of balance, Qi (universal energy) flows freely through pathways called meridians. The goal of Shiatsu is to facilitate an open flow of Qi by relieving any blockages that may occur from mental, emotional, nutritional or physical stresses and traumas.

Shiatsu is translated as finger pressure– shi (finger) and atsu (pressure). Typically, palms, elbows, fists, knees and feet are used as well. Traditionally, Shiatsu is performed on the floor. This allows practitioners to direct body weight more effectively and to easily use feet and knees, facilitating deeper work with less effort, wear and tear. Incorporating all applicable body parts as tools balances the demand on the practitioner's body, thereby reducing overuse of the hands and fingers.

The primary *technique* in Shiatsu is Compression. Effective compression is achieved by leaning and shifting body weight using gravity. The root source for this movement would be the Hara, the body's moving center (located below the naval). Though compression may be used 90% of the time there are other *techniques* incorporated at the discretion of the practitioner. They may include stretching, shaking, twisting, holding and even occasional pushing. All movement, for the most part, comes from the shifting of the Hara through the arms, hands, fingers, legs, feet, etc. Staying in touch with one's Hara is not only essential for good *body mechanics,* it also facilitates centeredness, which is vital to the process.

The practitioner becomes a conduit for energy when s/he establishes focused attention with a client and the tissue in the present moment. The nature of energy is that it wants to flow. A therapist simply remains open and present, allowing healing energy to move through. Sometimes doing less from a centered place can accomplish more. The dance of Shiatsu, like Tai Chi, is a moving meditation.

Shiatsu   # TouchAbilities®

Technique	Component	Skill
Compression	Compression	Pressing
	Breathing	Tracking, Pacing
Twisting	Compression	Twisting/Wringing
Stretching	Compression	Pushing
	Expansion	Pulling
	Gliding	Planing, Rubbing
Friction	Gliding	Planing, Rubbing
Shaking	Oscillation	Vibrating, Shaking
Tapotement	Oscillation	Striking
Traction	Kinetics	Mobilizing
Joint Rotation	Kinetics	Mobilizing

Deep Tissue Stone Massage

Bruce Baltz

Deep Tissue Healing, "the Art of Stone Massage" is the creation of Bruce Baltz. This approach works with intention, spiritual awareness and anatomical understanding in the application of natural stones. As therapeutic tools, stones are most commonly heated or chilled and can be used at neutral temperature. Whether used in a spa session or a medical treatment, they can serve as gliding pressure tools and/or as a source of thermal stimuli for the body. The efficient use of stones prevents strain on the therapists' hands.

Cold stones are hand-carved white marble; hot stones are basalt, river, or lava. The basalt stones are generally not cut, though they are often tumbled to make them more acceptable for *BodyWork*. Doing stone *massage* with the added benefit of temperature brings in healing properties that hands alone do not possess. Because the impact of the stones is amplified with temperature, knowledge of hydrotherapy principles involving the effects of heat and cold is essential.

Heat from the stones offers soothing, relaxing energy to release physical and mental stress and tight muscles. Cold is essential for balancing the treatment. It equalizes the natural heat inside the body, reduces the potential for discomfort and speeds the healing process. It is important to respect the therapist's tolerance and ability to handle heat as well as the client's tolerance for heat, cold and pressure. Less is often more.

Stones are more than just tools. Lava and marble stones can act as a bridge between spirit and the physical world. Holding the intention to create such a bridge, stones can ground both practitioner and client, creating the space for spiritual and emotional awareness. Working with stones is a very humbling experience, and in time they become one with the practitioner's hands and the work develops a *rhythm* all its own.

Deep Tissue Stone Massage

TouchAbilities®

Technique	Component	Skill
Pinning		
Palming	Compression	Pushing
	Gliding	Sliding
	Oscillation	Vibrating
Trailing Edge	Compression	Pressing
	Gliding	Sliding
	Oscillation	Vibrating
Cupping	Compression	Pressing
	Gliding	Planing
Claw Grip	Compression	Pressing
	Gliding	Planing
Palpating	Energetic	Sensing
Accepting Cold	Breathing	Directing

Hot Stone Massage

Ernesto Ortiz

Stones have been used throughout history for their capacity to hold and give energy. They have been employed for heating homes, making tools and sacred instruments as well as for healing. This particular approach is drawn from the traditions of the Lakota people.

Basalt stones, which come from lava, are the best to use because they hold heat and cold well. Using thermal stones is a powerful way to promote *homeostasis*, healing and balancing a person's physical, emotional, mental and spiritual aspects. Thermotherapy, the dynamic underlying principle of stone *massage*, is the application of either hot or cold stones to the body for the purpose of stimulating physiological responses. They produce a series of internal reactions including vasoconstriction and vasodilation. This, in turn, affects circulation and cellular nutrition, stimulates detoxification, relieves congestion and blockages in both muscles and visceral organs, and promotes healing. Alternating heat and cold during a treatment amplifies the effects of the work and produces what is called vascular gymnastics.

Treatments feature different stone placement patterns. Stationary stones are positioned on top of a towel, under a pillowcase or directly on the body. There are spinal layouts, front chakra layouts, special hand stones, cervical stones, etc. Some stones are used to glide on the body and some, like the hand stones, have a dual purpose– they can be stationary or used as *massage* tools.

Stones can be heated in a specially designed unit or an electric roaster with a thermometer for temperature control. For cooling, they can be kept in a small ice chest with ice packs or put in the freezer. Safety is very important, so attention to the temperature of the water and the stones, safety equipment for removing the stones, as well as thermal responsiveness of the client and therapist are critical.

Working with stones benefits both the client and the practitioner. When used effectively they reduce wear and tear on a therapist's hands, wrists and fingers. Some *indications* for stone *massage* are *acute inflammation*, sprains, strains, bursitis, *chronic* tension or just for pleasure. Clients come away with a deep meaningful connection to their body, having experienced new sensations, a profound sense of relaxation, openness to spirit, and a feeling of being totally pampered. Some claim to feel as delicious as melted chocolate.

Hot Stone Massage

TouchAbilities®

Technique	Component	Skill
Back Chakra Layout	Compression	Pressing
Front Chakra Layout	Compression	Pressing
Induction	Energetic Cognitive Breathing	Balancing, Intuiting Visualizing, Focusing, Transmitting Directing
Energy Connection	Energetic Cognitive Breathing	Balancing, Intuiting Visualizing, Focusing, Transmitting Directing
Stone Effleurage	Compression Gliding Oscillation	Pushing/Pressing, Squeezing Sliding Shaking
Hopi Technique	Energetic Cognitive Breathing	Balancing, Intuiting Visualizing, Focusing, Transmitting Directing
Tibetan Singing Bowl	Energetic	Sensing, Balancing

Swedish Massage

Mark Beck

Swedish Massage is currently the most common model for basic *BodyWork* in the United States. It denotes a relaxing, usually nonspecific, full body session using the traditional *techniques* of effleurage, petrissage, friction, tapotement and joint movements. Western therapeutic *BodyWork* has expanded and integrated the *techniques* of basic Swedish Massage to include *assessment* and planning procedures as well as a wider variety of *BodyWork techniques* such as compression, vibration and holding. Swedish Massage is directed mostly toward the physical body.

Receiving a Swedish Massage is a relaxing experience as the practitioner applies long, gliding strokes, squeezes and presses muscles and moves nearly every part of the client's body. Many of the *techniques* have either *direct*, mechanical effects on the soft tissue to which they are applied, or more *systemic*, reflexive effects that influence the autonomic nervous system. *Direct effects* include changes in *local* circulation, compression or stretching of muscle tissue and *fascia*. Effects to the autonomic nervous system may include stimulation of the sympathetic or parasympathetic nervous system, depending on the choice and duration of *BodyWork techniques*.

Basic Swedish Massage is often the first system of *BodyWork* a student is introduced to in school and is the most common treatment consumers expect when they make an appointment for *BodyWork* at a spa or clinic.

Swedish Massage

TouchAbilities®

Technique	Component	Skill
Touch	Kinetic	Holding
Effleurage/Gliding	Gliding	Sliding/Planing
Petrissage/Kneading	Compression	Pressing/Squeezing
	Expansion	Lifting, Rolling, Pulling
Friction	Compression	Pressing, Twisting/Wringing
	Gliding	Rubbing
Compression	Compression	Pressing
Vibration	Oscillation	Vibrating, Shaking
Tapotement/Percussion	Oscillation	Striking
Joint Movements	Kinetics	Mobilizing, Stabilizing
Assessment	Cognitive	Inquiring
Planning	Cognitive	Intending, Focusing

Traditional Thai Massage

Rose Griscom

Thai Massage is the physical *component* of an ancient holistic approach to healing the body/mind that has been practiced by monks within sacred temples throughout Thailand for over 1000 years (some say as much as 2500 years, since the coming of the Buddha in India and his follower, the Ayurvedic physician known throughout Southeast Asia as the Father Doctor *Shivago Komparpaj*). Traditional medicine encompassed manipulation (Thai Massage), application of herbs (topical and oral), nutrition/diet counseling, and spiritual practice (primarily expressed as vipassana meditation). Thai Massage or *Nuad Bo-Rarn* ("ancient healing way"), as it is commonly referred to in Thailand, focuses on the physical manipulation of the body, but the underlying principles incorporate aspects of Buddhism, Yoga, Ayurvedic Medicine, and Traditional Chinese Medicine.

In the Thai view, life force in the body travels along energy pathways known as *Sen* lines, which are broadly similar in theory and location to both traditional Chinese meridians and Ayurvedic nadis. It is believed that there is a direct correlation between physical and energetic imbalances expressed in the body. The therapist seeks to balance these energy pathways (and hence the whole body/mind) through manipulation of the musculoskeletal structure (compressing, pulling, lifting, twisting, supporting, shaking, stroking) sensing and affecting the muscles, *fascia*, joints, and energetic elements throughout the body.

Primary *techniques* are acupressure, compression and passive range of motion, coupled with conscious mindfulness, compassion and nonjudgment. The client remains comfortably clothed, lying on a floor mat, while the therapist proceeds through a systematic routine. Using his/her own body, assisted by leverage and gravity, the therapist carefully moves the client into a variety of stretches while simultaneously applying acupressure with the thumbs, palms, elbows or feet. With practice and seasoned knowledge, sessions become a flowing revitalizing dance guided more by intuition and energetic sensing than by a formal routine of movements.

Intended outcomes include physical changes such as softer connective tissue, lengthened muscle fibers, more space in the skeletal structure, reduced adhesions, increased circulation and lymphatic flow, deepened breath and revitalized internal organs. Emotional benefits are often experienced as calming, centering, with an increased feeling of comfort, joy and vitality. In this way, both the client and therapist can move together toward greater balance and a return to wholeness.

Traditional Thai Massage

TouchAbilities®

Technique	Component	Skill
Acupressure (with thumb)	Compression	Pressing
	Energetic	Sensing, Intuiting, Balancing
	Cognitive	Intending, Focusing
Rhythmic Compression (with thumb, palm, or foot)	Compression	Pressing
	Energetic	Balancing
Passive Range of Motion (stretching, tractioning, twisting, rotating)	Compression	Pushing, Twisting
	Expansion	Pulling, Lifting
	Kinetic	Holding/Supporting, Mobilizing, Stabilizing, Dropping/Letting Go
Rocking	Oscillation	Shaking
Chopping-Cupping-Rapping	Oscillation	Striking
Brushing	Gliding	Sliding
Forearm Rolling	Compression	Pressing, Pushing
Kneading	Compression	Squeezing
Pinching	Compression	Pinching
Circling (with thumb or palm)	Gliding	Planing, Rubbing
Breathing	Breathing	Tracking, Directing
Mindfulness & Connection	Cognitive	Inquiring, Intending, Focusing
	Energetic	Sensing, Intuiting, Balancing

Trager® Approach

Kathryn Hansman-Spice with
Byron Spice and Nan McConnaughy

The Trager® Approach is a form of movement re-education developed by Milton Trager, MD. It enhances function through tablework and Mentastics®, unstructured self-care movements which are guided by mental images and a process of inquiry. A core belief is that patterns are held in the unconscious mind and are changed when new feeling experiences offer new possibilities of well-being to the nervous system. New sensory information is needed to release unconscious holding patterns and to explore new patterns of moving, thinking and feeling that are more efficient and effortless.

In an alert, deeply relaxed, meditative *state*, described as "hook up," the practitioner acts as a facilitator, guiding the client into deeper self-awareness through gentle touch and movements. Working within the person's pain-free range, the practitioner engages in a process of sensing, acknowledging and asking without expecting specific outcomes. The practitioner listens with an attitude of acceptance and curiosity, heightening the client's awareness of sensations in the present moment. The key to effectiveness is an unconscious shift in attitude from effort to ease, without trying, using playful imagery and open-ended questions, such as "What could be lighter?"

If resistance is perceived, the practitioner does less to find the contact, position or movement that is most conducive to sending positive information to the unconscious mind. These passive movements create experiences of freedom, ease and natural fluidity for the client. If tone or functioning is diminished, Reflex Response is utilized to enliven and activate. The energetic effects of the treatment continue long after the session.

Mentastics® is utilized by practitioners and clients for their own self-renewal in order to be fully present in each moment. Clients are taught to Recall new awarenesses and possibilities in their daily lives through these playful, mindful movements, which either evolve from the session or are offered by the practitioner as tools of exploration for the client.

The Trager® Approach is a process, rather than a *technique*, which supports the natural healing powers of the body. The collaborative relationship between practitioner and client offers an invitation to new possibilities.

Trager® Approach

TouchAbilities®

Technique	Component	Skill
Psychophysical Integration	Cognitive	Visualizing, Inquiring, Focusing, Transmitting
	Energetic	Sensing, Intuiting, Balancing
Hook Up/Presence	Cognitive	Visualizing, Inquiring, Focusing, Transmitting
	Energetic	Sensing, Intuiting, Balancing
Mentastics® Movement Education	Cognitive	Visualizing, Inquiring, Focusing, Transmitting
	Kinetic	Holding/Supporting, Letting Go/Dropping, Mobilizing
	Oscillation	Vibrating, Shaking
Recall	Cognitive	Visualizing, Inquiring, Focusing, Transmitting
Process of Inquiry	Cognitive	Visualizing, Inquiring, Focusing, Transmitting
Reflex Response	Compression	Pressing/Pushing
	Breathing	Tracking, Directing
	Kinetic	Holding/Supporting, Mobilizing, Stabilizing Letting Go
Take Out the Slack/Extension	Expansion	Pulling
Joint Mobilization	Kinetics	Holding/Supporting, Mobilizing, Stabilizing Dropping/Letting Go
	Energetic	Sensing, Intuiting, Balancing
	Compression	Twisting
	Expansion	Pulling, Lifting, Rolling
Weighing	Expansion	Lifting
	Kinetic	Holding/Supporting
Compression	Compression	Pressing/Pushing, Squeezing
Sculpting	Gliding	Planing

Yamuna® Body Logic and Yamuna® Body Rolling

Yamuna Zake

Yamuna® Body Logic (YBL), created by Yamuna Zake, is a hands-on *modality*, that seeks to liberate the *body* on physical/structural, emotional/spiritual and energetic levels. The intention is to systematically free all muscle chains, reorganizing, educating and correcting structural issues that could be contributing to blockages/pain patterns and injuries. Even though a client may present with a specific injury or problem, the entire body is treated. This brings balance to the entire person, allowing the whole *body* to adapt, adjust and integrate any and all changes. YBL is done on the floor and the practitioner uses an elbow to work the target area, while the other hand applies traction. The entire *body* is worked by applying the traction with one hand while the elbow is used to work into the tractioned area.

Yamuna® Body Rolling (YBR) was created from the healing principles of Body Logic to empower people to take care of their own bodies. It is a healing self-massage technique that uses specially designed inflatable balls, 6-10 inches in diameter. The body bears down and rolls over the ball. Direct weight bearing into the ball stimulates bone and soft-tissue and stretches and elongates muscles from origin toward insertion. YBR is a tool for clients to use between sessions, for maintenance of current improvements and prevention from future injury.

There are five guiding principles of Body Logic and Body Rolling. The first is that the **Body has a Natural Logic and Order**. Where one muscle ends, another begins. Thus the work is done systematically through the connecting muscle groups. The key to repatterning is to see the muscles as a connecting chain and address a complaint in the context of the entire body. The next step is to identify how the client compensates and find out where that compensation begins in the muscles and tendons.

The second principle is that **Traction Creates Space**. In general, wherever there is restriction, compression, contraction, tightness, *inflammation*, atrophy or nerve pain, there is a lack of space. When a person experiences pain or discomfort due to sprain, muscle spasm, or nerve impingement, there is a compression or restriction in that specific area of the body. Creating optimum space throughout the body allows people their full range of motion in all joints and muscles.

The third principle is that of **Bone Stimulation**. YBL and YBR are done from the bone out. No matter what part of the body is focused on, the work begins with direct stimulation to the bone, then moves out into tendons and then into muscles. By applying direct pressure to a bone, any muscle that attaches anywhere on the bone begins to respond, releasing tension and elongating out from the bone.

The fourth principle relates to **Elongation of Muscles**. Working a muscle from its origin point with gentle traction toward its insertion provides optimal elongation of muscle.

The fifth principle involves the **Importance of the Spine**. The spine is considered the energetic and neurological life force of the *body*. Maintaining optimal alignment and length in the spine is essential for health. By minimizing spinal compression and maintaining healthy intervertebral space, the nerve roots are free and uncompressed. Energy is made accessible for the revitalization of all internal organs and the nervous system.

Function, movement, energy and emotional patterns will be restricted or blocked without a properly aligned structure. Both YBL and YBR seek to free the body of all restrictions on all levels – physical, emotional, mental and spiritual – so that each person can reach his/her desired human potential.

Yamuna® Body Logic

TouchAbilities®

Technique	Component	Skill
Traction	Kinetics Expansion	Mobilizing Pulling, Lifting
Bone Stimulation	Compression	Pushing/Pressing
Working Muscle from Bone into Tendon into Muscle	Compression Expansion Gliding	Pushing/Pressing Pulling, Rolling Planing
Range of Motion	Kinetics Compression Expansion	Mobilizing, Stabilizing Twisting Pulling, Lifting, Rolling
Gliding	Gliding	Sliding, Rubbing
Breath	Breathing Cognitive	Directing Focusing
Communication	Cognitive Energetic	Inquiring, Intending Sensing, Intuiting, Balancing
Weight Bearing	Compression Expansion Energetic	Pressing/Pushing Pulling, Rolling Sensing, Intuiting, Balancing

Yamuna®
Body Rolling

TouchAbilities®

Technique	Component	Skill
Traction	Compression	Pressing/Pushing
	Expansion	Pulling, Rolling
Cross Fiber Friction	Gliding	Sliding, Planing
	Compression	Pushing, Twisting/Wringing
Gliding	Gliding	Sliding, Planing, Rubbing
	Compression	Pressing/Pushing
Breath	Breathing	Directing
	Cognitive	Focusing, Transmitting
	Compression	Pressing
	Expansion	Pulling, Lifting

Zero Balancing

Fritz Smith

Zero Balancing (ZB) is a nondiagnostic system of healing which clarifies and coordinates energy *fields* in the body, and balances body energy with body structure. It is holistic and based on principles of nature. A typical session is done through clothing and lasts 30-45 minutes. A clear *state* of balance underlies health and happiness, and brings people closer to their true nature. Zero Balancing promotes this *state*.

ZB is a hands-on body/mind therapy that combines the Western view of science with an Eastern view of energy and healing. It is based on the quantum physics notion that the particle and the *wave* are the two fundamental aspects that comprise our universe and, in terms of the human being, comprise our structural and our energy bodies. Consciousness is the organizing principle that coordinates these foundations into one functioning whole and allows us to experience that process. Emotions are the vibratory frequencies that bring the process to awareness. ZB teaches that the deepest currents of energy are in bone, that memory is held in tissue, and that energy *fields* in the body underlie mind, body and emotions. Imbalances precede pathology. Hallmarks of ZB include focusing on the energetics of the bones and skeleton, guiding the treatment protocol by feedback signals, and working with expanded *states* of consciousness to clear *fields*.

Zero Balancing uses energy as its working tool in the form of a fulcrum. A fulcrum is a *field* of tension, which we create through touch. It serves as a catalyst to promote change and is itself not affected by its action. There are three, sometimes overlapping, classes of fulcrums: those that work as points of reference to promote balance and *local* change; those that work as *fields* to release less well-held vibration; and those that engage the client's own energy to promote change. The first group of fulcrums is held stationary for brief periods; the second group utilizes the form of a curve or, so-called half moon vector; the third group involves moving foci of energy. In all cases the fulcrum is performed at the interface of touch to ensure clear boundaries, and contacts both the body of energy and the body of structure.

Zero Balancing

TouchAbilities®

Technique	Component	Skill
Palpation/Objective (reading through touch)	Breathing	Tracking
	Energetic	Sensing
Evaluation for Held Energy (in soft tissue holding)	Kinetic	Mobilizing, Stabilizing, Supporting
	Energetic	Sensing
	Compression	Pushing
	Expansion	Pulling
	Breathing	Tracking
Evaluation for Ligament Tension & Joint Function	Kinetic	Mobilizing, Stabilizing, Holding/Supporting
	Compression	Pushing/Pressing
	Expansion	Pulling
	Breathing	Tracking
	Energetic	Sensing
Fulcrum as Reference Point (stationary)	Kinetic	Holding
	Compression	Twisting/Wringing
	Expansion	Lifting, Pulling
	Breathing	Tracking
	Energetic	Sensing
Fulcrum to Promote Local Change (stationary)	Compression	Twisting/Wringing
	Expansion	Pulling, Lifting
	Breathing	Tracking
	Energetic	Sensing
Fulcrum for Field Effect (curved tension)	Kinetic	Mobilizing
	Compression	Pressing, Twisting
	Expansion	Pulling, Lifting
	Breathing	Tracking
	Energetic	Sensing

Zero Balancing
(continued)

TouchAbilities®

Technique	Component	Skill
Fulcrum as Moving Engagement of Energy Bolus	Compression	Pushing/Pressing
	Expansion	Pulling
	Breathing	Tracking
	Energetic	Sensing
	Gliding	Planing

"A massage therapist touches and rubs the tissue, a[n] herbalist applies an extract of a plant, an acupuncturist applies a needle, magnet, electrical stimulation or laser beam, a Shiatsu practitioner applies deep pressure, a practitioner of the Rolf technique stretches a layer of fascia, a sound therapist vibrates the tissue, a medical doctor uses a pulsating electromagnetic field, etc. The common denominator in all of these approaches is a living matrix that is exquisitely designed to absorb the information encoded in different kinds of vibratory energy and convert it into signals that are readily transmitted through the tensegrous semiconducting living matrix continuum."

Jim Oschman, PhD,
The Journal of Bodywork
and Movement Therapies,
January 1998, 2(1), pg. 55

Conclusion

Our *body* is a gift and our responsibility. This intelligent *multidimensional* structure houses our essence and carries us through the world. We, alone, are in the position to care for and maintain optimal function of this *body* in order to enjoy a long and healthy life.

To accomplish this, we must consciously tune in to the inherent signs and signals that provide information about our *states* of being. By creatively using TouchAbilities®, we can uncover the mystery, wonder and awe of the *body*. In the pursuit of balance and good health, TouchAbilities® provides tools for self-care and support of others.

The concept of TouchAbilities® establishes basic elements of intra/interpersonal connections through *BodyWork*. It presents an indivisible, unified whole that is arbitrarily divided to allow for flexible and creative comprehension and application. In the realm of *body*, nothing exists alone; everything is connected.

"Our perspective values self-responsibility, authentic self-exploration, self-expression and the healing relationship.... This means the individual person plays an active responsible role in his or her healing and preventive healthcare.... Practitioners... will be a valuable resource to individuals who are actively engaged in composing their lives, defining their personal visions of health, and learning from and responding to life's adventures."

Elliot Dacher,
Noetic Sciences Review,
Summer 1997,
No. 42, pg.14

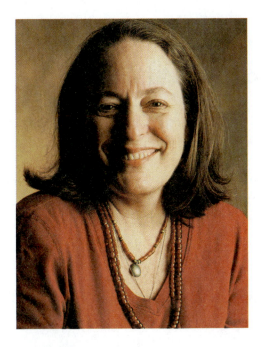

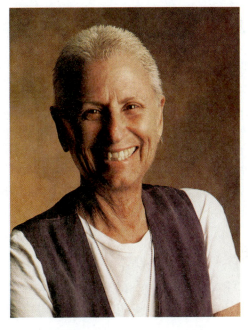

Iris Burman
Educating Hands School of Massage
120 SW 8th Street
Miami, Fl 33130
305-285-6991 ● 1-800-999-6991
iris@touchabilities.com

Sandy Friedland
Bayview Plaza
1621 Bay Road #707
Miami Beach, Fl 33139
305-546-4178
sandy@touchabilities.com

If you are enthusiastic about the ideas presented in this book and would like to explore other TouchAbilities® projects and products, log onto our website: **www.touchabilities.com**. You will find information regarding seminars, teacher training, curriculum development and implementation, as well as personal and group coaching.

Let us know how this book affects your life and the lives of those you touch.

In touch,

Iris and Sandy

TouchAbilities®
Practitioner's Actions Synopsis

Use this section as a practical guide to the physical actions involved in performing the TouchAbilities® skills. When we refer to the *body* we mean the multidimensional dynamic of *body*, mind, emotion and spirit of both the client and the practitioner. When we say, "place whatever *body* part you're using on the target area of the client's *body*" it encompasses physical, emotional, mental and spiritual domains (PEMS). Our use of the term *target area* also reflects the PEMS realms.

Breathing Component

TRACKING- Employ your senses of touch, sight, smell and hearing to notice the client's pattern of inhalation and exhalation.

DIRECTING- Use your own breath, physical contact and/or verbal communication to influence the client's breathing cycle.

PACING- Adjust your breathing cycle and/or other *BodyWork* applications to match the client's breathing cycle.

Cognitive Component

VISUALIZING- Hold a mental image in your own mind and/or have the client do the same.

INQUIRING- Use your thought mechanisms and/or verbal skills to seek an answer to a query and/or have the client do the same.

INTENDING- Use your mind to consciously create a plan or purpose and/or have the client do the same.

FOCUSING- Use and aim your conscious awareness at a target and/or have the client do the same.

TRANSMITTING- Use your mental power to send a signal toward a goal and/or have the client do the same.

Energetic Component

SENSING- Use your innate biological mechanisms (sight, touch, smell, hearing, taste, proprioception, etc.) to experience internal and external stimuli.

INTUITING- Allow yourself to tap into wisdom emerging from your unconscious.

BALANCING- Use whatever skills and capacities you have to influence your client's dynamic nature in the direction of homeostasis.

Compression Component

PRESSING- Place whatever *body* part/s you're using on the target area of the client's *body*. Stay in one place and lean down into that location using your own *body* weight.

PUSHING- Place whatever *body* part/s you're using on the target area of the client's *body*. Lean, using your own *body* weight to produce movement away from the original point of contact.

SQUEEZING- Place any two of your own *body* parts on opposite sides of the client's target area and move them toward each other.

PINCHING- Place the tips of your fingers and thumbs on opposite sides of your client's target area and move them toward each other.

TWISTING- Use your hands to grasp some point on the client's *body* (either the target area itself or some location in relation to the target area) and apply a turning motion.

WRINGING- Place your hands on two points of a client's target area, compress and move them toward and past each other.

Expansion Component

PULLING- Use your hands to grasp some point on the client's *body* (either the target area itself or some location in relation to the target area) and lean your *body* away from the client's *body*.

LIFTING- Place whatever *body* part/s you're using under the target area of the client's *body* and lift. One can also lift a target sructure by grasping from above and lifting up.

ROLLING- Place your hands on the target area of the client's *body*. Squeeze and lift some skin or tissue between your fingers and thumb. Maintaining the lift, roll the tissue by moving your hands in a continuous forward or backward motion. To travel and create momentum, that is, to keep the tissue rolling, your lead digits walk and your following digits scoop under the roll and lift and move in coordination with the lead digits.

Kinetics Component

HOLDING- Place whatever *body* part/s you're using onto the target area of the client's *body* and maintain a static contact.

SUPPORTING- Place whatever *body* part/s you're using under the target area of the client's *body* and exert sufficient effort to bear the weight of the target area.

MOBILIZING

    ACTIVE- Instruct the client to move his/her own *body* part/s at joint/s.

    PASSIVE- Take hold of and move the client's *body* part/s at joint/s. (In this instance, the client makes no effort.)

LETTING GO- Release the contact between your *body* part/s and those of your client.

DROPPING- From a raised position, remove and release your support of the client's *body*.

STABILIZING- Place whatever *body* part/s you are using against one side of a target joint on the client's *body* and exert sufficient effort to limit movement.

Oscillation Component

VIBRATING- Place whatever *body* part/s you're using on the target area of the client's *body* and apply tremulous, *rhythmic* motion.

SHAKING- Place whatever *body* part/s you're using on the target area of the client's *body* and move it *rhythmically* side to side or back and forth.

STRIKING- Use part/s of your own *body* (most commonly hands) to make intermittent and broken contact to the target area of your client's *body*.

Gliding Component

SLIDING- Place whatever *body* part/s you're using on the target area of the client's *body*. Glide on/over the surface of the target area.

PLANING- Place whatever *body* part/s you're using on the target area of the client's *body*. Glide along any of the subcutaneous layers of tissue. Compress with sufficient effort to engage the target strata or to move through descending levels of tissue.

RUBBING- Place whatever *body* part/s you're using on the target area of the client's *body*. Move back and forth, diagonally or circularly over that surface area, creating friction. For subsurface or deeper layers of tissue, marry your *body* part/s to the surface tissue and slide this layer back and forth, diagonally or circularly over underlying tissue.

Hand Exercises

Doing these "handy maneuvers" on a regular basis will keep your body, especially your back, arms and hands, strong and flexible. For starters, do each exercise 10 times for each hand, then build up to more repetitions. Remember that hand care and palpatory sensitivity are vital elements of being a powerful practitioner.

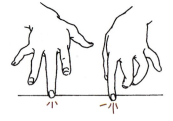

Hold your hands in front of your chest and shake them briskly enough to get them warm and loose.

Hold a small ball, some putty, or clench your hand into a tight fist. Squeeze the ball, putty or your fist as hard as you can and hold. Repeatedly doing this exercise can strengthen your hands and wrists.

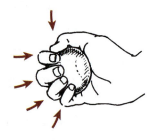

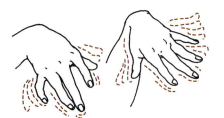

Place both hands palms down on a flat surface. Tap each finger—moving from thumb to pinky and back again— as if you were playing the piano or typing. Practice this kind of tapping to improve your coordination and hand control.

Place your palms together in front of your chest. Press one hand against the other and go back and forth. Repeating these presses can make your wrists supple and strong.

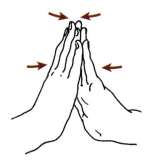

Begin at your thumb and massage all the fingers of your hand by rubbing each of them from the metacarpal-phalangeal joint to the distal tip. Regularly massaging your fingers this way can stimulate circulation and keep them supple.

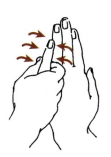

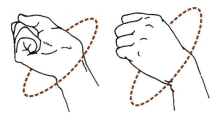

Make a fist and rotate your hand in circles in front of you. Going clockwise and counterclockwise with each hand— in both directions— can keep your wrists and forearms strong and flexible.

As you press the fist of one hand into the palm of the other have them resist each other. Pressing back and forth this way can strengthen your hands and arms.

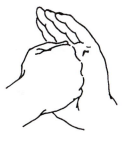

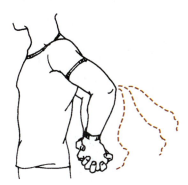

Clasp your hands behind your back just below your waist. As you maintain the tension, slowly pull your arms up, then slowly push your arms down. Doing this exercise can strengthen your arm, shoulder and hand muscles.

Research Citations

1. Beeken, J. E., & Parks, D. (1998). Effectiveness of neuromuscular release massage therapy. *Clinical Nursing Research*, 7: 309.

2. Fakouri, C., & Jones, P. (Feb 1987). Relaxation Rx: Slow stroke back rub. *Journal of Gerontological Nursing*, 13 (2), 32-35.

3. Ferrell-Torry, A. T. & Glick, O. J. (Apr 1993). The use of therapeutic massage as a nursing intervention to modify anxiety and the perception of cancer pain. *Cancer Nursing*, 16 (2), 93-101.

4. Meek, S. S. (Spring 1993). Effects of slow stroke back massage on relaxation in hospice clients. *Journal of Nursing Scholarship*, 25 (1), 17-21.

5. Danneskiold-Samsoe, B., Christiansen, E. & Anderson, R. B. (1986). Myofascial pain and the role myoglobin. *Scandinavian Journal of Rheumatology* (Stockholm), 15, 174-78.

6. Weintraub, M. (Apr 1992). Shiatsu, Swedish muscle massage and trigger point suppression in spinal pain syndrome. *American Journal of Pain Management*, 2 (2), 74-78.

7. Hammer, W. I. (1993). The use of transverse friction massage in the management of chronic bursitis of the hip and shoulder. *Journal of Manipulation & Physical Therapeutics*, 16(2), 107-111.

8. Smith, L. L., et al. (Feb 1994). The effects of athletic massage on delayed onset muscle soreness, creatine kinase, and neutrophil count: A preliminary report. *Journal of Orthopaedic & Sports Physical Therapy*, (2), 93-99.

9. Sunshine, W., Field, T., et al. (Feb 1996). Fibromyalgia benefits from massage therapy and transcutaneous electrical stimulation. *Journal of Clinical Rheumatology*, 2(1), 18-22.

10. Weintraub, M. (Apr 1992). Shiatsu, Swedish muscle massage and trigger point suppression in spinal pain syndrome. *American Journal of Pain Management*, 2 (2), 74-78.

11. Baumann, J. U. (1996). Effect of manual medicine in the treatment of cerebral palsy. *Manuelle Medizin* (Berlin), 34, 127-133.

12. Cady, S. H., & Jones, G. E. (Feb 1997). Massage therapy as a workplace intervention for reduction of stress. *Perceptual & Motor Skills*, 84(1), 157-158.

13. Fakouri, C., & Jones, P. (Feb 1987). Relaxation Rx: Slow stroke back rub. *Journal of Gerontological Nursing*, 13 (2), 32-35.

14. Meek, S. S. (Spring 1993). Effects of slow stroke back massage on relaxation in hospice clients. *Journal of Nursing Scholarship*, 25 (1), 17-21.

15. Curtis, M. (Sept 21-27, 1994). The use of massage in restoring cardiac rhythm. *Nursing Times* (England), 90 (38), 36-37.

16. Meek, S. S. (Spring 1993). Effects of slow stroke back massage on relaxation in hospice clients. *Journal of Nursing Scholarship* 25 (1), 17-21.

17. Baumann, J. U. (1996). Effect of manual medicine in the treatment of cerebral palsy. *Manuelle Medizin* (Berlin), 34, 127-133.

18. Kaada, B. & Torsteinbo, O. (1989). Increase of plasma beta endorphins in a connective tissue massage. *General Pharmacology*, 20 (4), 487-89.

19. Jensen, O. K., Neilsen, F. F., Vosmar, L. (Oct 1990). An open study comparing manual therapy with the use of cold packs in the treatment of post-traumatic headache. *Cephalalgia* (Norway), 10 (5), 241-50.

20. Puustjarvi, K., Airaksinen, O., & Pontinen, P. J. (1990). The effects of massage in patients with chronic tension headache. *Acupuncture & Electro-Therapeutics Research*, 15 (2), 159-62.

21. Shulman, K. R., & Jones, G. E. (June 1996). The effectiveness of massage therapy intervention on reducing anxiety in the workplace. *The Journal of Applied Behavioral Science*, 32(2), 160-173.

22. Wilkinson, S. (Jan/Mar 1995). Aromatherapy and massage in palliative care. *International Journal of Palliative. Nursing*, 1 (1), 21-30.

23. Ferrell-Torry, A. T., & Glick, O. J. (Apr 1993). The use of therapeutic massage as a nursing intervention to modify anxiety and the perception of cancer pain. *Cancer Nursing*, 16 (2), 93-101.

24. Drinker, C. K., & Yoffey, J. M. (1941). Lymphatics, lymph and lymphoid tissue: Their physiological and clinical significance. *Cambridge: Harvard University Press.*

25. Elkins, E. C., Herrick, J. F., & Grindlay, J. H., et. al. (1953). Effects of various procedures on the flow of lymph. *Archives of Physical Medicine and Rehabilitation,* 34, 31.

26. Mortimer, P. S., Simmonds, R., & Rezvani, M., et.al. (1990). The measurement of skin lymph flow isotope clearance - reliability, reproducibility, injection dynamics, and the effect of massage. *Journal of Investigative Dermatology,* 95, 766-682.

27. Badger, C. (1986). The Swollen Limb. *Nursing Times (England),* 82 (31): 40-41.

28. Bunce, I. H., Mirolo, B. R., Hennessy, J. M., et al. (1994). Post-mastectomy lymphedema treatment and measurement. *Medical Journal of Australia,* 161, 125-28.

29. Zanolla, R., Monzeglio, C., Balzarini, A., et al. (1984). Evaluation of the results of three different methods of postmastectomy lymphedema treatment. *Journal of Surgical Oncology,* 26, 210-13.

30. Field, T., Hernandez-Reif, M., & Ironson, G. (1998). Massage therapy effects on breast cancer *(unpublished).*

31. Ironson, G., Field, T., et al. (1996). Massage therapy is associated with enhancement of the immune system's cytotoxic capacity. *International Journal of Neuroscience,* 84, 205-217.

32. Zeitlin, D., et al. (Jan/Feb 2000). Immunological effects of massage therapy during academic stress. *Psychosomatic Medicine,* 62, 83-87.

33. Meek, S. S. (Spring 1993). Effects of slow stroke back massage on relaxation in hospice clients. *Journal Nursing Scholarship,* 25 (1), 17-21.

34. Field, T., Peck, M., Hernandez-Reif, M., Stern, S., Burman, I., Krugman, S., & Ozment-Schenck, L. (2000). Postburn itching, pain, and psychological symptoms are reduced with massage therapy. *Journal of Burn Care and Rehabilitation,* 21, 189-193.

35. Field, T., Peck, M., Krugman, S., Tuchel, T., Schanberg, S., Kuhn, C., & Burman, I. (1997). Burn injuries benefit from massage therapy. *Journal of Burn Care and Rehabilitation,* 19, 241-244.

36. Hernandez-Reif, M., Field, T., Largie, S., Hart, S., Redzepi, M., Nierenberg, B., & Peck, M. (2001). Children's distress during burn treatment is reduced by massage therapy. *Journal of Burn Care and Rehabilitation,* 22, 191-195.

37. Field, T., Hernandez-Reif, et al. (1997). Labor pain is reduced by massage therapy. *Journal of Psychosomatic Obstetrics and Gynecology,* 18, 286-291.

38. Dundee, J. W., Sourial, F. B., Ghaly, R. G. & Bell, P. F. (Aug 1988). P6 Acupressure Reduces Morning Sickness. *Journal of Royal Society of Medicine,* 81 (8), 456-57.

39. Culpepper-Richards, K., (July 1998). Effect of a back massage and relaxation intervention on sleep in critically ill patients. *American Journal of Critical. Care,* 7(4), 288-299.

Research References

Web Links to Research Studies

http://nccam.nih.gov
(NCCAM *Manual Therapies*)

www.internethealthlibrary.com

www.massagetherapyfoundation.org

www.miami.edu

www.intelihealth.com
(*Harvard Medical Schools consumer health information on massage*)

www.amtamassage.org
(*back pain*)

www.vancouvermassage.ca

www.massagemag.com
(*compilation of research articles from the magazine*)

www.holistic-online.com
(*enter: massage research*)

www.petmassage.com

www.clinicaltrials.gov

www.nlmta.ca
(*back pain*)

www.ncbi.nlm.nih.gov
(*links to studies on various topics*)

Books About the Research Process

Domholdt, E. (2000). <u>Physical therapy research</u>. (2nd ed). Toronto: Saunders.

Menard, M. (2003). <u>Making sense of research</u>. Toronto: Curties-Overzet Publications.

Hagino, C. (2001). <u>How to appraise research: A guide for chiropractic students and practitioners</u>. London: Churchill-Livingston.

Rich, G. J. (Ed). (2002). <u>Massage therapy: The evidence for practice</u>. Edinburgh: Mosby.

Peters, D. (Ed). (2001). <u>Understanding the placebo effect in complementary medicine</u>. London: Churchill-Livingstone.

Hymel, G. (2005). <u>Research methods for massage and holistic therapies</u>. Edinburgh: Mosby.

References

Benjamin, B. (2004). Follow the principles of ergonomics. *Massage Therapy Journal*, 43:1: 30-33.

Blackburn, J. (2003). Table-talk: Verbal interaction – The missing piece in bodywork. *www.jackblackburn.homestead.com/articlesbyjack.html*.

Chaitow, L. (1991). Palpatory literacy. Hammersmith, London, England: Thorsens.

Chopra, D. (1995). The way of the wizard. New York, NY: Harmony Books.

Dacher E. (1997). Healing values: What matters in health care. *Noetic Sciences Review*, 42: 10-17.

Ford, C. (1989). Where healing waters meet : Touching the mind and emotions through the body. New York, NY: Talman Company.

Goldman J. (1996). Healing sounds: the power of harmonics. Boston, MA: Element Books Limited.

Harman, W. (1998). Global mind change...The promise of the 21st century. San Francisco, CA: Berrett-Koehler Publishers, Inc.,

Juhan, D. (1995). Somatic explorations. *Massage Magazine*, No. 54: 56-63.

Kabat-Zinn, J. (1994). Wherever you go, there you are. New York, NY: Hyperion.

Keleman, S. (1986). Bonding. Berkeley, CA: Center Press.

Keleman, S. (1985). Emotional anatomy. Berkeley, CA: Center Press.

Keleman, S. (1975). Your body speaks its mind. Berkeley, CA: Center Press.

Knaster, M. (1996). Discovering the body's wisdom. New York, NY: Bantam Books.

Kroeger, H. (2002). Help one another. Boulder, CO: Hanna Kroeger Publications.

Lauterstein, D. (1998). The mind in bodywork. *Massage Therapy Journal*, 37:3: 108-111.

Lauterstein, D. (1997). Breath and the coming of age of energywork. *Massage Therapy Journal*, 36:2: 119-122.

Leape, L. (February 2003). Florida reducing medical errors. *www.nursingceu.com*.

Lordi, J. (2003). Taichi and its applications for massage therapy. *Massage Therapy Journal*, 42:2: 45-52.

MacPherson, H. (1994). Body palpation and diagnosis. *Journal of Chinese Medicine*, 44:1: 1-7.

Martin Nicolas. (2002). *American Iatrogenic Association*, www.iatrogenic.org.

McDonough T. (1998). The energy fascia connection. *Massage Magazine* No. 73: 2-99.

McPartland, JM. (1998). Cranial osteopathy and craniosacral therapy: Current opinions. *The Journal of BodyWork and Movement Therapies*, 2:1: 29-31.

Milne H. (1995). The heart of listening 1; A visionary approach to craniosacral work: Origins destination points, unfoldment. Berkeley, CA: North Atlantic Books.

Milne, H. (1998). The heart of listening 2: A visionary approach to craniosacral work: Anatomy, technique, transcendence. Berkeley, CA: North Atlantic Books.

Myers T. (2000). A language revolution. Massage Magazine, No. 85: 20-22.

Myers T. (2004). The star of depth. Massage & BodyWork, xix:4: 88-95.

Myss, C. (2003). Intuition and the mystical life (CD w/ Clarissa Pinkola Estes). Boulder, CO: Sounds True Audio.

Naparstek, B. (2000). Intuition, imagery & healing seminar brochure.

Naparstek, B. (2005). www.conferenceworks.com.

Null, G., Dean, C., Feldman, M., Rasio, D. (Nov. 2003). Death by medicine-8, www.garynull.com.

(Aug. 1998). Reducing healthcare error: Systems-based approaches and nursing perspectives. Nursing World/Nursing Trends & Issues; Vol 3, No. 8, www.nursingworld.org.

Oschman J. (1997). What is healing energy: The scientific basis of energy medicine - Part 5A. Journal of Bodywork and Movement Therapies 1(5): 297-309.

Oschman J. (1997). What is healing energy: The scientific basis of energy medicine - Part 6. Journal of Bodywork and Movement Therapies 2(1): 46-60.

Palmer, H. (1994). Resurfacing®...techniques for exploring consciousness. Altamonte Springs, FL: Star's Edge® International.

Palmer, P. (1998). The courage to teach: Exploring the inner landscape of a teacher's life. San Francisco, CA: Jossey-Bass, Inc.

Shea, M. (1998). The art of teaching touch: Theory and practice of adult learning and development. Juno Beach, FL: Shea Educational Group, Inc.

Shea, M. (1996). Somatic psychology for bodyWorkers. Juno Beach, FL: Shea Educational Group, Inc.

Smith, FF. (1986). Inner bridges: A guide to energy movement and body structure. Atlanta, GA: Humanics Publishing Group.

Stephens, R. (2002). Beyond the rub, Massage Today, 2:9.

Tolle, R. (2005). The trager approach, Massage Therapy Journal, 44:1: 61-67.

(1986). Webster's third new international dictionary. Springfield, MA: Merriam-Webster, Inc.

Werner, A. (2005). A massage therapist's guide to pathology. Baltimore, MD: Lippincott Williams & Wilkins.

Practice Errors Resources

Agency for Health Care Administration (AHCA)
www.fdhc.state.fl.us

Agency for Healthcare Research and Quality (AHRQ)
www.ahrq.gov

Herbal information for relationship with other medications
www.herbs.org

Joint Commission on Accreditation of Healthcare Organizations
www.jcaho.org

Physicians Desk Reference
www.pdr.net

Institute for Safe Medication Practices
www.ismp.org

National Center for Patient Safety
www.patientsafety.org

Professional Organizations

There are many professional BodyWork organizations. They provide support, status, education, cama-raderie, leadership opportunities, buying power, lobbying power and networking to practitioners. Two professional organizations that cater to the broadest spectrum of BodyWorkers and massage therapists are the AMTA, which is focused, but not limited to, Western techniques and the AOBTA, which is focused on Eastern techniques. Many individual modalities have established organizations that represent their specialized interests. To reference these groups refer to the listings in Massage Magazine.

AMTA
American Massage Therapy Association
500 Davis Street, Suite 900
Evanston, IL 60201
877-905-2700 toll free
847-864-0123 local
847-864-1178 fax
www.amtamassage.org

AOBTA
American Organization for Bodywork Therapies of Asia
1010 Haddonfield–Berlin Road, Suite 408
Voorhees, NJ 08043
856-782-1616 local
856-782-1653 fax
www.aobta.org

Publications

The following periodicals feature editorials and articles on research, modalities and trends in the field. Some may include product and seminar advertising, listings of conventions, articles on business development, practice management and legislative updates. They discuss the issues facing the profession and present personal stories and experiences. All are available by subscription and most are available at newsstands and in bookstores.

Massage Magazine
5150 Palm Valley Road, Suite 103
Ponte Vedra, FL 32082
800-533-4263 toll free
904-285-6020 local
904-285-9944 fax
www.massagemag.com

> Massage Magazine includes a regular listing of the associations for the various modalities, reports the latest guidelines for licensure in the states that regulate massage and provides a resource directory of schools.

Massage Therapy Journal
500 Davis Street, Suite 900
Evanston, IL 60201
877-905-2700 toll free
847-864-0123 local
847-864-1178 fax
www.amtamassage.org

> Massage Therapy Journal is the publication of the American Massage Therapy Association (AMTA) and can be subscribed to independent of membership. It features listings of schools that are COMTA accredited.

Journal of Bodywork and Movement Therapies
Elsevier Journals Customer Service
6277 Sea Harbor Drive
Orlando, FL 32887
877-839-7126 toll free
407-345-4020 local
407-363-1354 fax
www.harcourt-international.com

> The Journal of Bodywork and Movement Therapies is the only academic peer review publication for the BodyWork and movement professions. It has no advertisement other than for its own yearly conference and features editorials, peer reviewed articles, technique papers and strategies for working with practical issues in musculoskeletal function, treatment and rehabilitation. This is available only through subscription.

Massage and Bodywork
c/o ABMP
1271 Sugarbush Drive
Evergreen, CO 80439
800-458-2267 toll free
303-674-8478 local
800-667-8260 fax
www.abmp.com

> Massage and Bodywork Magazine is a publication of the Associated Bodywork and Massage Professionals, a private, for-profit group that offers insurance and networking opportunities for massage therapists.

Regulatory Agencies

COMTA
Commission on Massage Training Accreditation
1007 Church Street, Suite 302
Evanston, IL 60201
847-869-5039 local
847-869-6739 fax
www.comta.org

> COMTA is the accrediting agency for schools of massage and BodyWork. As a regulatory organization, its purpose is to set entry-level standards for massage education and ensure that a school accredited by them meets specific criteria. To become accredited, each school must comply with a stringent set of standards aligned with the guidelines of the U.S. Department of Education. The Commission is comprised of nine elected members. They meet twice a year to consider new applicants and oversee and review issues that pertain to currently accredited schools. COMTA status provides assurance for the prospective student that a school has met these standards

NCBTMB
National Certification Board of Therapeutic Massage and Bodywork
8201 Greensboro Drive, Suite 300
McClean, VA 22102
800-296-0664 toll free
703-610-9015 local
703-610-9005 fax
www.ncbtmb.com

> NCBTMB is the certifying agency for individual therapists. This board sets minimum competency standards for the practice of professional massage therapy. To become certified a therapist must complete approved educational programs and pass a national exam. NCBTMB certification status supports the therapist, because it signifies professionalism and credibility.

Training and Certification

Basic BodyWork education in the United States is available in every state, but the length, depth, quality and focus vary greatly. For the most part, professional level training is presented in 500-1000 hours and includes studies in anatomy, physiology, pathology, basic massage techniques and hygienic practice. In addition, some schools provide classes in hydrotherapy, business development, personal growth and introductions to specific modalities. Many schools have some form of clinic where students work with the general public to practice their developing skills. The foundational skills as taught in most schools today are based in Swedish style techniques. Globally it is the most widely recognized form of massage by both recipients and employers. In the United States, over the last 25-30 years, there has been an infusion of many styles of BodyWork from other parts of the world, particularly from the Far East and Europe. The field is thriving with innovation. Practitioners have created new approaches or introduced variations on old approaches that are now recognized modalities. Today, there are many entry-level schools that present a modality other than Swedish as their base curriculum, such as Shiatsu, Pfrimmer, NMT, Polarity, etc. In these schools the BodyWork philosophy is geared to that particular modality and specific techniques are stressed that support their special focus. Minimum education requirements vary from state to state. In the U.S. they range from 250 hours required in Texas to 1000 hours required in Nebraska and New York. As of this writing, the most common state requirement throughout the country is 500 hours.

Acute– critical, serious, in need of urgent care; extremely sharp or intense; a condition in which the signs and symptoms begin abruptly with marked intensity and subside in a short period of time; an intensification phase of an ongoing, *chronic* condition. (see *Chronic*)

Adaptation– the process or *state* of changing to fit new circumstances or conditions, or the resulting change; diminished response of a sense organ to a sustained stimulus; modification of an organism or its parts that makes it more fit for existence under current conditions.

Adverse event– an injury or death resulting from health care management, not from the underlying condition of the patient. (see *Error*)

Affirmation– a positive statement, made in the present tense, stating something as if already true; to establish and affirm an intention or goal; to imagine that something is already so programs the unconscious mind to achieve that goal.

Autoimmunity– a condition in which the *body's* immune response acts against its own tissues; determined by genetic influences as well as environmental triggers; causes a broad range of human illnesses, known collectively as autoimmune diseases.

Assessment– the systematic process of gathering information in order to make informed choices; in relation to *BodyWork*, it may involve client history, observation, palpation and other evaluative procedures.

Body– an intricate *multidimensional* complex of systems and energy *fields* associated with an organism including and extending beyond the physical plane; incorporates physical, mental, emotional and spiritual essence integrating anatomy, physiology and energy; a living form that is defined and animated by its amorphous, ever-changing energetic nature and the vibrating, pulsating, dynamic mechanisms of its physicality.

Body Mechanics– the use of energy and physical structure in the performance of a task; "Good" *body mechanics* is an art, a seamless flow of combinations of posture, balance, direction, locomotion, stillness, strength, intention and angle.

BodyView– a *general* approach through which to "see" a *body*. (see *Modality*)
- Energetic View
- Functional View
- Movement View
- Structural View
- Convergent View

BodyWork– as a **profession**, *BodyWork* is characterized by the collection of systems, *modalities*, designed to interact with the *body* in support of balance and good health; as an **action**, it is the *skillful*, intentional application of the *techniques* of any of the *modalities* within the profession. (see *Modality*)

Boundary– the real or imagined edge, limit or extent of something; a line, plane or edge representing a physical, emotional, mental or spiritual border that determines the limits of something.

Carrier Wave– a *wave* or current whose modulations are used to carry signals through and between *bodies*.

Chronic– a condition that persists or recurs over a long period of time; slowly progressing intensification; marked by long duration or frequent recurrence. (see *Acute*)

Cognitive– the act or process of being aware, knowing, thinking, learning and judging; knowing by the use of reasoning, intuition or perception– including such things as analysis, application, awareness, comprehension, synthesis, evaluation and meta-cognition.

Component– a part or element of a larger whole.

Contact Point– the points of the practitioner's *body*, such as hands, feet, elbows, forearms, knees, etc., through which power is transmitted to and received from the client's *body*. (see *Ground Point*)

Contagious– easily diffused or spread from one person to another; relating to communicable diseases; capable of being transmitted by infection; spread by direct or indirect contact between people or organisms.

Contraindication– a symptom or particular circumstance that leads a therapist to cautiously apply or refrain from applying a therapeutic procedure; metaphorically, this translates to a "yellow light" for caution and a "red light" for avoidance. (see *Indication*)

Contralateral– originating in or affecting the opposite side of the *body*. (see *Ipsilateral*)

Countertransference– a projection of therapist's feelings and other personal life issues on to the client. (see *Transference*)

Direct Effect– the initial consequence of an application of mechanical or energetic forces; happening concurrent with and as a result of the interaction between the therapist and the client. (Also referred to as **primary**, **mechanical**). (see *Indirect Effect*)

Domain– a distinctly defined sphere of knowledge or activity; one's peculiar and exclusive function or *field* of active cultivation and responsibility.

Endangerment Site– physical locations of the *body* that are especially vulnerable, delicate or exposed; involves tissues and structures such as nerves, blood vessels, organs and lymph nodes unprotected by bone, muscle or connective tissue that can be in danger from pinching, pinning, occluding or entrapment.

Entrainment– being in step or in synch with; matching; mutual attraction and reciprocal response; the ability of a strong rhythmic vibration to cause a less powerful rhythmic vibration to synchronize with it. (see *Resonance*)

Ergonomics– the study of designing objects to be better adapted to the shape of the human *body* and/or to correct the user's posture; an applied science concerned with designing and arranging things people use so that the people and things interact efficiently and safely; the study of how a workplace and the equipment used there can best be designed for comfort, safety, efficiency and productivity.

Error– an occurrence that is viewed as problematic: execution error– failure of a planned action to be completed as intended; thought or planning error– use of a wrong plan to achieve an aim; equipment error– involving poor quality, inferior maintenance or unskilled usage leading to a problem. (see *Adverse Event*)

Eustress– positive, normal, healthy stress that stimulates learning, growth and integration. (see *Stressors*)

Fascia– thin, elastic connective tissue that forms an uninterrupted *multidimensional* network from head to foot; a fibrous membrane covering, supporting, separating every muscle, bone, nerve, gland, organ and blood vessel in the *body*.

Facilitated Pathway– a neural response pattern embedded in the nervous system by repetition associated with a learned activity.

Feedback Loop– a cycle of mutual interaction in which each agent responds to the other's actions; a circuit of communication and feedback involving output and input, sending and receiving.

Field– a realm of forces in dynamic interplay; a coherent realm with identifiable qualities and specific characteristics.

Field of Engagement– an interpersonal *field* established between beings; a place of interfacing edges; the connection between individuals where the composite elements of their *bodies* interact.

General– affecting the entire *body*; applicable to, involving or affecting the whole. (see *Local*, *Regional* and *Systemic*)

Ground Point– in *body mechanics*, the place from which power is created; the place of origin/the starting point of an action or the root of a *wave*; the stable points from which to originate and generate power to be transmitted to the client. (see *Contact Point*)

Holarchy– an order of increasing holons, of increasing wholeness and integrative capacity. A principle popularized in the cosmology of holistic philosopher Ken Wilber meaning "everything is simultaneously a part of something larger than itself (a higher whole), and a whole in its own right is made up of its own smaller parts. Everything is a holon, in the sense that it is a whole in one context, and a part in another."

Homeostasis– the balance within the internal environment of the *body* (microcosm) and the dynamic relationship between the *body* and the external environment (macrocosm).

Iatrogenic– a negative reaction to medical treatment or therapy which is a result of the treatment itself and not due to the underlying condition; any adverse condition, e.g., harm, disease, illness, or death, resulting from treatment by a health care practitioner; an abnormal state or condition induced by a health care practitioner or by medical treatment or diagnostic procedures.

Immunosuppression– suppression of or interference with the *body's* immune response. It may reflect natural immunologic unresponsiveness (tolerance); may be deliberate, i.e., artificially induced by chemical, biological or physical agents (e.g., medication for patients receiving organ transplants); may be incidental (as a side effect of radiotherapy or chemotherapy for cancer); or could be caused by disease (e.g., HIV). Decreased immune response increases the *body's* susceptibility to infectious disease.

Indication– a symptom/signal or particular circumstance that supports the necessity for a therapeutic procedure; metaphorically, *indications* are "green lights" to apply *techniques* in response to a specific aspect of a client's condition. (see *Contraindication*)

Indirect Effect– the multifaceted physiological and psychological response to a *direct* application. This application sets into motion a series of reactions, which continue to affect the *body* over time at various levels (physical, emotional, mental, spiritual) and in various locations, sometimes other than that of the initial connection. These reactions are ongoing ripple *effects* of the original application. (Also referred to as **secondary** or **reflex**.) (see *Direct Effect*)

Inflammation– a protective response of *body* tissues to injury, infection, irritation or disease; characterized by pain, swelling, redness and heat, sometimes leads to loss of function; a mechanism initiating elimination of noxious agents and damaged tissues.

Ipsilateral– on the same side; affecting the same side of the *body*. (see *Contralateral*)

Kinetics– a branch of dynamics that deals with the effects of forces upon the motions of material bodies (Webster's 3rd New International Dictionary); an umbrella term for a collection of *skills* that focus on the movement relationship between segments of the *body*.

Local– a restricted place, part or area of the *body*; pertaining to one spot or location. (see *General*, *Regional* and *Systemic*)

Malpractice– the act or failure to act by a member of the health care professions that results in harm, injury, distress, prolonged physical or mental suffering or death.

Mantra– an expression or idea that is repeated often, to transform consciousness.

Massage– skillful manipulation of soft tissue, connective tissue and/or *body* energy *fields* with the intention of maintaining or improving health by affecting change in relaxation, circulation, nerve responses or patterns of energy flow. (from the AMTA – American Massage Therapy Association – *Scope of Practice*). (see *BodyWork*)

Mastery– competence, proficiency, the possession of profound knowledge; a combination of *skill*, wisdom and expertise; a level of excellence; high-level integration of *skill*, focus and strategy.

MDMA®– an acronym for Multi-Dimensional Movement Arts®, a *modality* developed by Sandy Friedland that utilizes *waves* and pulses in the application of touch *skills*, performed in a water environment.

Modality– the method of application of a therapeutic agent or regimen; a system comprised of a selection and organization of touch *skills*, based on a particular viewpoint or organizing principle, applied to a *body* to effect an intended outcome. *Modalities* include a variety of philosophical approaches, theoretical frameworks, and specific combinations of *skills*. (see *BodyWork* and *BodyView*)

Mobility– the capacity for and facility of movement.

Motility– the capacity for spontaneous but unconscious or involuntary movement (Mosby's Medical Dictionary); the vital *wave* of life that animates tissue.

Multidimensional– relating to or marked by several dimensions. (A dimension is a level of consciousness, existence or reality); a unit comprised of quantities, qualities, aspects and variables.

Palpation– feeling or perceiving through the senses

Paradigm– a shared set of assumptions; a fundamental, basic way of perceiving, thinking, valuing and doing, associated with a particular view of the world; a pattern or model for something, especially one that forms the basis of a methodology or theory.

Presence– a *state* of attention and awareness that is mindful and alert and "in the moment."

Projection– attributing one's own feelings, ideas, attitudes to other people or objects; unconscious transfer of a personal thought, feeling, or impulse to somebody else.

Proprioception– the ability to receive stimuli produced within our own *body*; "the awareness of posture, movement and changes in equilibrium and the knowledge of position, weight and resistance of objects in relation to one's own *body*." (Webster's 3rd New International Dictionary).

Proprioceptive Neuromuscular Facilitation (PNF)– specific *techniques* that activate the *body's* own "receptors" to shift muscle tone, promote relaxation and support lengthening.

Regional– related or limited to a particular region/characteristic of an area; a particular area or part of the *body*. (see *Local, General* and *Systemic*)

Resonance– the frequency at which an object most naturally vibrates (bones, tissues, organs and every other part of the *body* have a specific resonant frequency); vibrations of one vibrating *body* reach out and influence the vibrations of another *body*. (see *Entrainment*)

Rhythm– harmonious or orderly movement, fluctuation or variation; a pattern of elements suggesting movement or pace in something or any regularly recurring pattern of activity or repeated functions of the *body*.

Scope of Practice– the range of activities included in a given profession; may be determined by legislation, education, interest and *skill* development, life experiences, size, endurance, etc.

SenseAbilities™– a variety of possible sense experiences; a context for sensations that might be experienced when engaged in *BodyWork*; a sense vocabulary to define experience and promote awareness.

Severe– a condition that is harsh, intense, serious, difficult, extremely strong or powerful; intensely or extremely bad or unpleasant in degree or quality or extent, causing pain, difficulty, anxiety, damage, etc.

Skill/s– proficiency, facility, or dexterity that is acquired or developed through training or experience; the basic core elements of TouchAbilities®; the fundamental ways in which people can interact with each other; can be applied individually but are more usually combined with each other to create specialized *techniques*. (see *Technique*)

S.O.A.P. – an acronym for subjective, objective, *assessment* and plan. These words are categories within a system for charting findings and treatment progress notes.

State– the status, mode or condition of being; a condition or stage in the physical constitution of something.

Stressors– stimuli or agents that elicit a response from the *body*; an activity, experience or situation that causes stress.

Systemic– affecting the whole; affecting an entire *body* system or the *body* as a whole; involving physiological, psychological or energetic systems in their individual function or in the way they interface with each other. (see *General, Local and Regional*)

Technique– a method, procedure, process, way or manner used to accomplish a desired aim; in TouchAbilities®, *technique* refers to a *skill* or combination of *skills* blended and used simultaneously to support an intended outcome.

Thixotropy (thixotropic)– a structural property of certain substances to liquefy when subjected to vibratory forces, heat or other energy influences, and to solidify again when left standing; a material that gels when stationary and liquefies when agitated. Everyday examples: toothpaste, ketchup, mustard.

Tensegrity or "tensional integrity"– a property of objects with *components* that use tension and compression in a combination that yields strength and resilience beyond the sum of their parts; synergy between co-existing pairs of fundamental physical laws such as push/pull, compression/tension, or repulsion/attraction.

Toning– a system of healing that uses the human voice to resonate different areas of your own, or another person's *body*; vocal sounds used to alter vibrations in every molecule and cell in the *body*.

TouchAbilities®– the fundamental ways of interacting with and/or acting upon and between *bodies*. These "ways" are foundational or seminal to the development of *Modalities*.

Trajectory– a path, projection or line of transmission.

Trajectory of Force– an imagined pathway between therapist and client on which power, energy and information can be sent and received.

Transference– displacement of feelings toward someone or something else; client projects family or intimate relationship patterns of feelings and behaviors onto the therapist, i.e., behaving toward the practitioner as if they were their father, mother or spouse. (see *Countertransference*)

Wave– a rolling or undulating movement or one of a series of such movements passing along the surface of, or through matter in all its forms.